A Course in Intensive Therapy Nursing

A Course in Intensive Therapy Nursing

Jack Tinker BSc MB ChB MRCP FRCS DIC

Director of the Intensive Therapy Unit
The Middlesex Hospital
London

Susan W Porter SRN ONC

Nursing Officer
Intensive Therapy Unit
The Middlesex Hospital
London

Edward Arnold
A division of Hodder & Stoughton
LONDON MELBOURNE AUCKLAND

First published in Great Britain 1980
Reprinted 1985, 1988, 1991

British Library Cataloguing in Publication Data

Tinker, Jack
A course in intensive therapy nursing.
1. Critical care medicine
2. Intensive care nursing
I. Title II. Porter, Susan W
616 RC86.7

ISBN 0-7131-4347-9

Typeset in V.I.P Century Schoolbook by Western Printing Services Ltd, Bristol. Printed and bound in Great Britain for Edward Arnold, a division of Hodder and Stoughton Limited, Mill Road, Dunton Green, Sevenoaks, Kent TN13 2YA by J. W. Arrowsmith Ltd, Bristol

Preface

The care of critically ill patients demands the highest standards of nursing care and skill. Nurses wishing to work in the specialized field of intensive therapy must, accordingly, undertake a substantial, practical and theoretical, programme of training. In England and Wales the Joint Board of Clinical Nursing Studies have outlined a curriculum for a six-month post-registration course in general intensive care nursing.

This book has been written with the aims of this, and other intensive therapy training programmes, in mind. It is primarily intended for nurses wishing to specialize in intensive therapy, but we hope that nurses working in related fields and those in training will also find it to be of help.

London, 1980

JT
SWP

Acknowledgements

We wish to acknowledge the unstinting help of Julie Ray, Shobhna Shah and Sonia Crossley in the preparation of this book; also to thank Miss Sara Morgan and Miss Pamela Hibbs for their helpful comments and the many other colleagues who have advised and criticized.

We are grateful to Mr Paul Darton, Mrs Ann Burns and Miss Diana McLean for preparing the illustrations and Mr Eric Leung for his photographic help.

Contents

1

Introduction

Critical illness disturbs in varying degrees the function of the major physiological systems: cardiovascular, respiratory, renal—electrolyte and neurological. At the onset usually one system is predominantly affected but, as the disturbance progresses, others become involved. For example, the circulatory failure of an extensive myocardial infarction may lead to respiratory and renal failure, whilst the respiratory failure of severe pneumonia may lead to cardiac and then renal failure. An appreciation of this pattern of close inter-relationships between the body systems is central to the management of critical illness for, irrespective of its initial cause, it presents fundamentally similar problems that constitute the foundation of intensive therapy.

Historically, intensive therapy has arisen by the integration of a number of originally separate disciplines. As different methods of assessing and managing critically ill patients became available, units appeared that were named according to the special service they offered: respiratory units for ventilation, renal units for dialysis and coronary care units for cardiac monitoring are all familiar examples. However, because of the many similarities referred to, all critically ill patients can be effectively managed in integrated, general intensive therapy units (ITUs). It is now both unnecessary and uneconomic to have a multiplicity of individual units in a single hospital.

Selection of patients for intensive therapy

The selection of patients for intensive therapy is of fundamental importance.

An ITU provides many services, ranging, from a detailed observation of vital signs to the total support of failing physiological systems and, as a general rule, patients requiring any or all of these facilities should be considered for admission. Patterns of admission, however, vary from one unit to another depending on the workload of the hospital, the availability of staff and the level of care that can be provided on the general wards. From an economic standpoint the bed occupancy in a unit should be kept near a maximum. Most ITUs operate optimally with an overall occupancy of between 75 and 80 per cent, but even at this level the stresses and strains on the staff and equipment can be considerable.

Specific criteria for selection do therefore differ from one unit to another but there are a number of general considerations which serve as helpful guidelines.

The illness must be judged to be reversible; an ITU is certainly not the place for the care of patients in the terminal phases of chronic disease. Acute-on-chronic illness, however, presents a very difficult problem, for often even if the acute phase is reversible the patient will only be restored to a state of permanent disablement. Patients should not be admitted solely for 'heavy nursing'—a euphemism which usually implies a number of intractable problems that are not in any way immediately life-threatening.

The age of the patient is a necessary consideration, but old age should never be the sole reason for refusing admission if other criteria are fulfilled.

A relatively high mortality rate (usually between 10 and 30 per cent) is inherent in the nature of the work but it must not be compounded by inappropriate patient selection. If this happens the morale of the staff declines, many leave and recruitment becomes difficult.

The intensive therapy unit

The number of beds allocated for an ITU is related to the size and work of the hospital. A common ratio is one ITU bed for every 100 acute beds, with an additional one or two if the hospital has a cardiothoracic or neurosurgical department. Units having less than six beds are uneconomic whilst those with more than 12 are difficult to manage; eight is an optimum number. This means that small hospitals cannot economically support an ITU, and poses the problem of organizing intensive therapy on a regional basis.

Within the hospital the ITU should be readily accessible from the accident and emergency department, the operating theatres and the general wards. Such a location can be planned for when designing new hospitals but in older ones the choice of site often represents a compromise. Wherever its situation, the planners must try to ensure that the unit will be light and spacious, for this vastly improves working conditions and minimizes the patients's sense of isolation.

In the unit the beds may be arranged either in an open-plan or in separate rooms. At least two rooms have to be provided for the isolation of infected cases. Indeed, there are many advantages for having all of the beds in individual rooms: then the noise level in the unit is reduced, the chances for cross-infection are minimized and fully conscious patients are protected from the disturbing atmosphere of a busy ITU. The only disadvantage of such an arrangement is the extra demand it can make for numbers of nursing staff, so often some combination of both is adopted.

The unit also requires a large storage area, a staff room, sleeping accommodation for the doctor on duty, a laboratory and a room for the patients' visitors (Fig. 1.1).

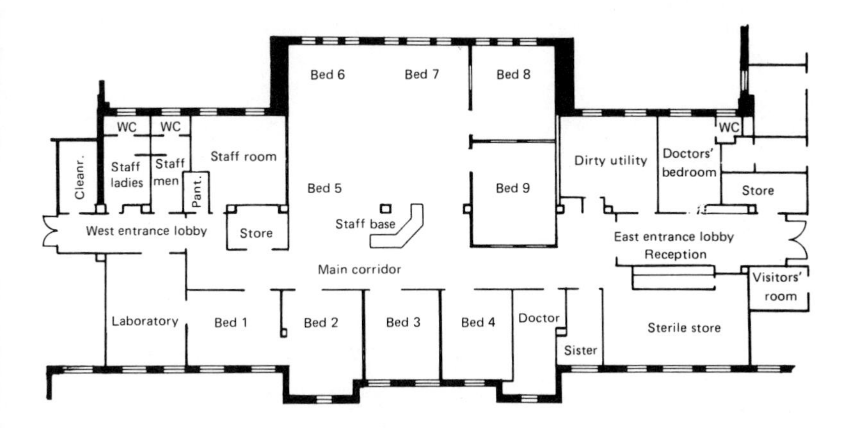

Fig. 1.1 A plan of the Middlesex Hospital ITU.

Services and equipment

Intensive therapy requires a large number of engineering services and many kinds of equipment. Technical services must be adequate and the number of electrical sockets at each bed head should be sufficient for all the equipment that might be in use; between eight and 12 are needed. Piped oxygen compressed air and suction are vital, and outlets for each are required on either side of the bed head. The range of equipment used varies widely depending on the unit but certain items of monitoring, respiratory and resuscitative equipment are essential. These can be all mounted conveniently on a wall rail behind each bed (Fig. 1.2).

Monitoring

There should be provision at each bed for continuous electrocardiographic monitoring and measurement of central venous pressure with a saline manometer. Heart rate meters and alarms are helpful if used properly. Electronic methods for the direct measurement of arterial and venous pressures are certainly useful but need skilled technical help. In an ITU, where a nurse is usually required to be constantly at the bedside, a central monitoring station has limited value.

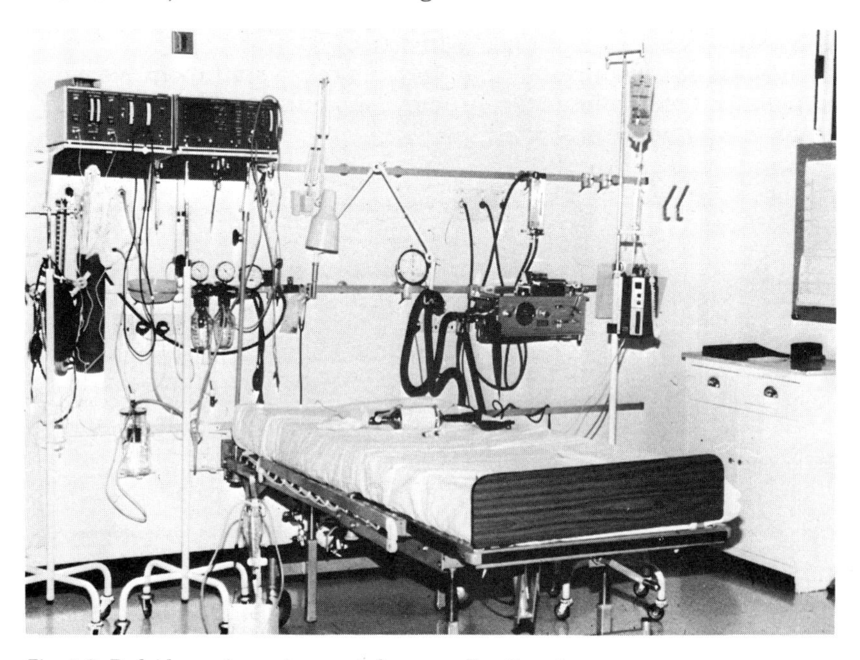

Fig. 1.2. Bedside equipment mounted on a wall rail system.

Respiratory

Ample equipment for oxygen therapy, humidification of inspired gases, suction and mechanical ventilation is essential.

Resuscitation

Emergency cardiorespiratory resuscitation is an important component of intensive therapy. Equipment for defibrillation, hand ventilation and intubation must always be immediately available.

Staff

Nursing

Intensive patient care is totally dependent on the availability of sufficient numbers of trained nursing staff. Because the patients need continuous care, staffing is based on a formula of one nurse per patient for each 24 hours—a quota of approximately 4.25 nurses per bed. Most will be staff nurses with special training or experience in intensive therapy.

Because of the specialized nature of intensive therapy nursing, the Joint Board of Clinical Nursing Studies have detailed the curriculum for six-month post-registration courses. Furthermore, the grouping of critically ill patients in a single unit means that nurses working in the general wards no longer gain experience in their management. This has important implications for students in training and they should spend some time in an ITU preferably during their final year.

Nurses working in an ITU experience a variety of stresses, some of which are inevitable, due to the very nature of the work. All the patients are seriously ill and many are unconscious, delirious or unable to communicate. The rapid rate of patient turnover and close contact with death result in frequent separations and re-attachments. Distressed and highly anxious relatives have to be managed firmly but with great compassion. The nurse carries responsibility for the interpretation of rapidly changing physical signs, understanding the behaviour of equipment and, from time to time, initiating emergency resuscitation. Although many of the problems are inseparable from the situation of dealing with severely ill patients they must nevertheless be recognized and can, in most instances, be ameliorated by an empathic nursing administration and efficient medical organization.

Medical

It is regrettable that the organization of medical staffing for an ITU is still often unsatisfactory. A unit must have its own medical staff to co-ordinate and implement patient care. Intensive therapy is currently emerging, albeit slowly, as a distinct specialty, and as more people are trained in this field the situation will improve.

Technical

The work of supervising, maintaining and using the large amount of equipment requires a full-time physiological measurement technician who will also be responsible for blood gas and electrolyte analysis.

Physiotherapy

Physiotherapists carry out a great deal of respiratory therapy in addition to the general physiotherapy. An ITU should have on its staff a qualified physiotherapist with special training in intensive therapy.

Cost

Intensive therapy, because of the large numbers of trained staff required and, to a lesser extent, the amount of equipment used, is expensive. The daily cost per patient has been estimated to be four or five times that of a patient on a general ward. Such high costs have inevitably invited questions on the ethics of concentrating so much of the resources on a relatively small number of patients. Unquestionably the development of ITUs in the past decade has saved many lives and has greatly improved the level of efficiency of care offered to critically ill patients. It has also influenced the standards of nursing and medical care generally. The cost is well recognized but any reductions will have a profound effect on patient care and survival.

Section A
Physiology

2

Cardiovascular physiology

Anatomy

Certain important anatomial features of the heart and major vessels are shown in Fig. 2.1.

Functionally the heart can be considered as two separate pumps, a right and a left, which are arranged in series and circulate the blood from the venae cavae through the pulmonary and systemic circulations. The ventricles are the important pumping elements; at rest the atria function mainly as reservoirs but in exercise their contraction contributes to the increase in cardiac output.

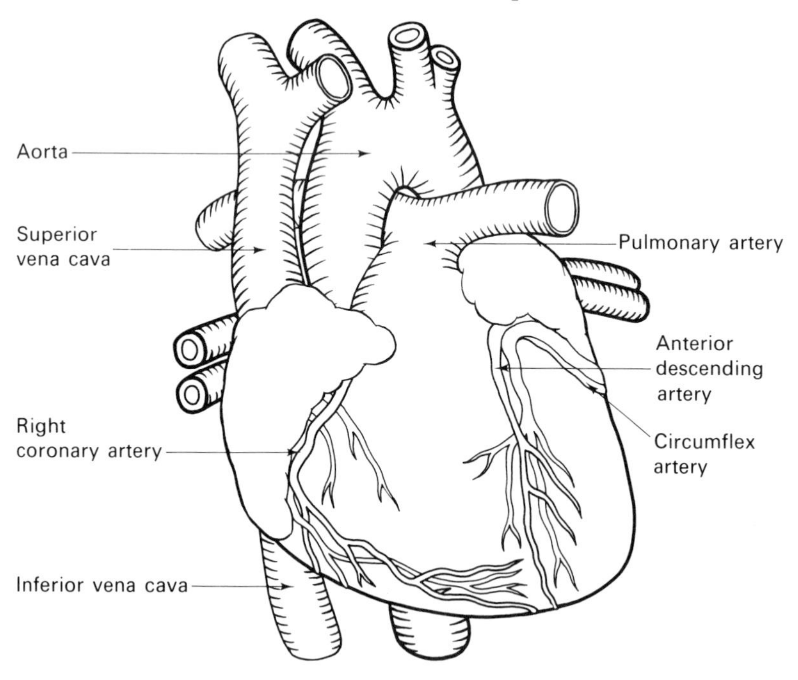

Fig. 2.1 Cardiovascular anatomy.

Valves are positioned at the inflow and outflow of each ventricular chamber to ensure a unidirectional flow of blood.

Within the chest the heart lies inside the pericardial sac which completely invests it together with the origins of the great vessels. The pericardium has two layers: a thin visceral one, attached to the surface of the heart, and a thicker outer parietal one. The two are normally separated from each other by a small quantity of pericardial fluid.

The coronary circulation

Two coronary arteries, a right and a left, supply oxygenated blood to the myocardium. They originate from the root of the ascending aorta, just above the aortic valve, and pass in opposite directions along the atrioventricular groove (Fig. 2.1.).

The right coronary artery supplies branches to the right atrium and ventricle; it also supplies the atrioventricular (AV) node and, in approximately 60 per cent of individuals, the sinoatrial (SA) node. On the inferior surface of the heart it gives off the posterior descending branch and then anastomoses with a branch of the left coronary artery.

The left coronary artery divides, soon after its origin, into an anterior descending and a left circumflex branch. The circumflex branch passes along the atrioventricular groove to the inferior surface of the heart and supplies the left atrium and ventricle and the SA node where this is not supplied by the right coronary artery. The anterior descending branch courses downwards in the anterior interventricular groove and supplies the ventricular septum and left ventricle.

The coronary venous return is via a number of veins draining into the coronary sinus which opens into the right atrium near the tricuspid valve.

Radiology

Portable chest x-rays are frequently used in the assessment and management of patients in an ITU (Fig. 2.2.). They permit evaluation of the heart, pulmonary vasculature and lung fields, and are essential for locating the position of central venous or other intracardiac catheters, or pacemaker wires.

The heart shadow is seen in contrast to the relatively translucent lung fields; its transverse diameter is normally less than half the total width of the chest. The right border of the cardiac silhouette is formed by the superior vena cava and the right atrium. On the left side, the upper part is formed by the arch of the aorta, below which are the pulmonary artery and its left main branch. The remainder of the left border consists of a small segment of the left atrium followed by the left ventricle which also forms the apex of the heart.

Interpretation of a portable chest x-ray requires careful and systematic inspection of the film. Because they are often taken under difficult circumstances they may not be properly aligned and the image of the various structures will then be distorted, making interpretation difficult.

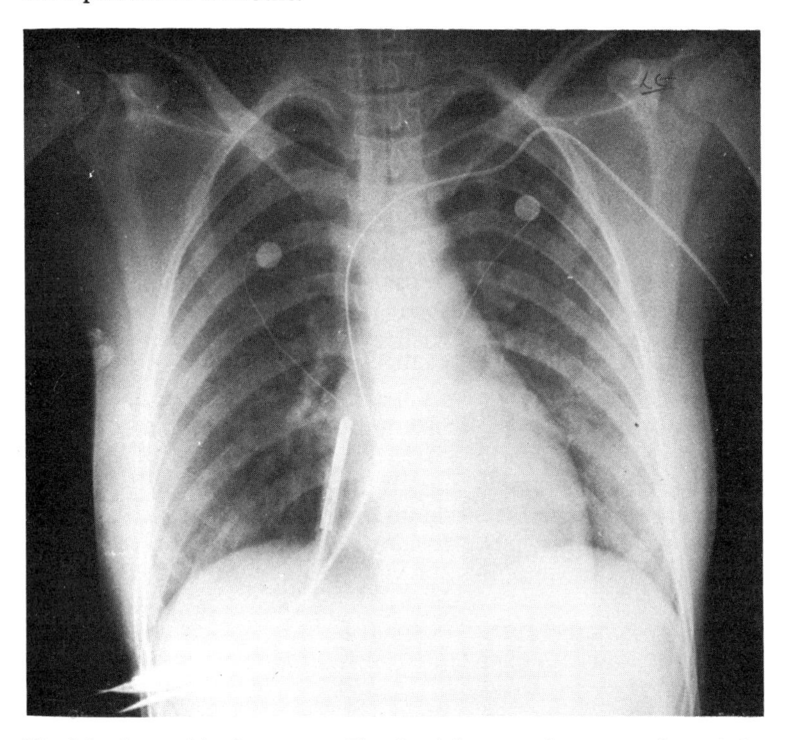

Fig. 2.2 A portable chest x-ray: The tip of the central venous catheter is located in the right atrium and the tip of the endotracheal tube is above the carina. The end of the nasogastric tube is visible in the stomach.

The conducting system of the heart

Certain cells in the heart have the special function of initiating and conducting the electrical impulses that are responsible for muscle contraction. They are grouped into a number of defined structures: the sinoatrial (SA) node, the atrioventricular (AV) node, the bundle of His and its right and left bundle branches (Fig. 2.3.).

The SA node is the pacemaker of the heart and its rate of impulse formation determines the heart rate. It is situated in the wall of the right atrium at the junction with the superior vena cava. The impulses originating from it are conducted across the atrial muscle to the AV node, a localized structure in the floor of the right atrium that constitutes the sole 'communications' link between the atria and the ventricles. After passage through the AV node they are conducted through the bundle of His and its right and left bundle branches to the Purkinje network, the ramification of small conducting fibres that finally lead to the ventricular muscle cells.

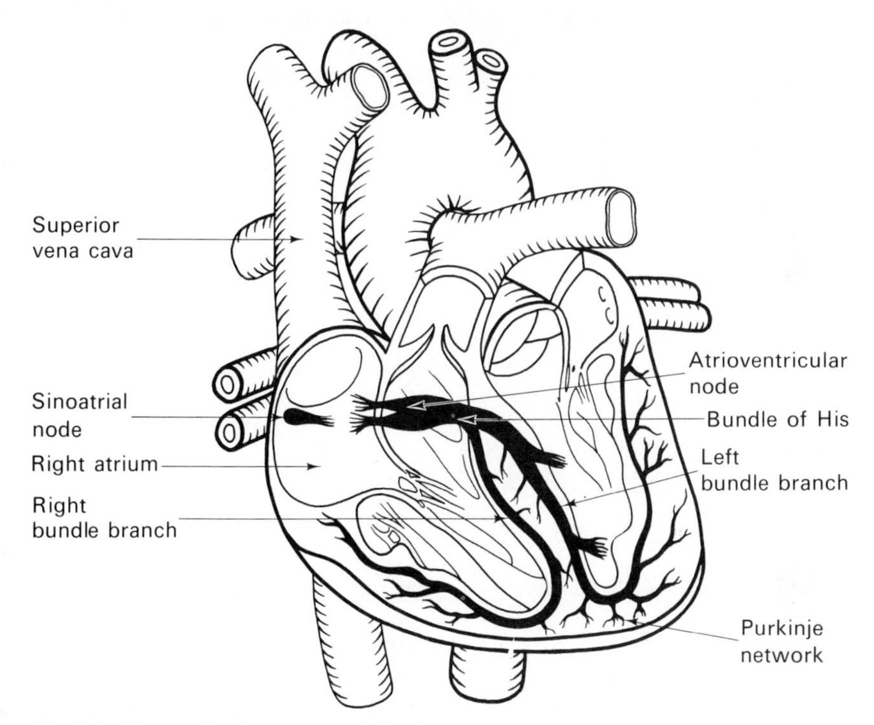

Fig. 2.3 The conducting system of the heart.

The SA node is supplied by both the sympathetic and the parasympathetic divisions of the autonomic nervous system, and the heart rate, at any one time, reflects the balance of activity between each of these components. Increase in the sympathetic activity increases heart rate, whilst an increase in parasympathetic activity decreases it. The parasympathetic supply to the heart is through the vagus nerve and its inhibitory effect is often referred to as 'vagal tone'.

The actions of the sympathetic nerves are mediated by the liberation of adrenaline and noradrenaline at the nerve endings and are augmented by the release of these same compounds from the adrenal medulla; acetylcholine is the transmitter substance liberated from the parasympathetic nerve endings. The overall level of autonomic activity on the heart is reflexly governed from the cardiac centre in the brain stem.

Divisions of the sympathetic nervous system

The sympathetic nervous system is functionally divided into alpha and beta components, a separation that has major therapeutic implications for the use of a large number of cardiovascular drugs. The beta sympathetic is further subdivided into beta 1 and beta 2 elements. The heart is supplied by beta 1 endings and the bronchi and skeletal muscle arterioles by beta 2. All the other arterioles are supplied by the alpha division.

Stimulation of the beta 1 sympathetic causes an increase in heart rate and force of cardiac contraction whilst stimulation of the beta 2 endings produces bronchial, and skeletal muscle arteriolar, dilatation. Stimulation of the alpha sympathetic results in widespread arteriolar constriction and an increase in peripheral resistance. Isoprenaline mimics the action of the beta 1 and 2 sympathetic systems (sympathomimetic), and beta-blocking drugs such as propranolol and oxprenolol, as the term implies, block their action, the latter being selective for beta 1 endings. Noradrenaline stimulates the alpha endings, and alpha-blocking drugs such as phenoxybenzamine and phentolamine block their effect.

The actions of the parasympathetic nerves are blocked by atropine.

Electrical events of the cardiac cycle

In the resting state each heart muscle cell has a positive electrical charge on its surface and a negative charge inside; it is therefore said to be polarized. During contraction this charge is lost (depolarization) and is regained during recovery (repolarization).

The nett electrical changes stemming from the depolarization and repolarization of all heart muscle cells form the basis of the electrocardiogram (ECG). Since the body acts as an electrical conductor, these changes, although reduced in magnitude, can be detected on the skin surface.

The normal electrocardiogram

A typical ECG complex is shown in Fig. 2.4. It signifies the electrical changes, recorded in millivolts (mV), occurring during the time of one cardiac cycle; the five main deflections are designated P, Q, R, S and T.

The P wave relates to atrial depolarization and is of low amplitude in comparison with the other deflections.

The P–R interval is the time period, measured from the beginning of the P wave to the beginning of the QRS complex, including both the P wave and the P–R segment. It therefore represents the time taken for the impulse to pass from the SA node to the ventricles. Normally it measures less than 0.2 second and longer times than this imply a delay in conduction, most often in the AV node.

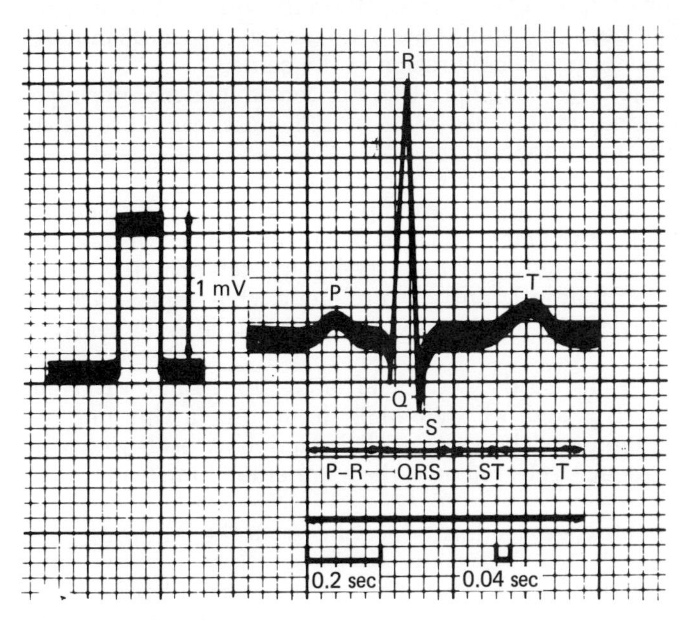

Fig.2.4 A normal ECG complex.

The QRS complex originates from depolarization of the ventricular muscle cells. It has an initial negative Q wave, followed by a positive R wave, and then a negative S wave. The amplitude of each particular wave depends to a large extent on the position of the recording electrodes in relation to the heart, and sometimes one or other may not be present. Nevertheless, the same rules of nomenclature apply. The Q wave is always the first negative deflection, the R wave the first positive, and the S wave is the negative deflection that follows an R wave.

The S–T segment is the period between the S and T waves and is part of ventricular repolarization.

The T wave represents ventricular repolarization and in the normal ECG is always positive.

For purposes of analysis the ECG waveform can be divided into two sections: one, consisting of the P wave and P–R segment, that represents supraventricular events and the other, the QRST, that is related to ventricular activity. Such a division provides a most convenient and practical method of classifying and interpreting the cardiac dysrhythmias.

Measurements. Standard ECG recordings are made at a paper speed of 25 mm per second so that, on the recording paper, each large square equals 0.2 second and each small one 0.04 second (Fig. 2.4). The vertical deflections of the ECG represent electrical voltages, the standard calibration being two large (10 small) squares to one millivolt (1 mV). On monitor displays the trace also sweeps at 25 mm per second and the amplitude calibration is the same.

Lead systems for recording the ECG. For continuous monitoring of the ECG the signal is obtained via a single chest lead (three electrodes) but in the standard record twelve leads are used (Fig. 2.5)—six from the limbs and six from the chest.

The standard leads (I, II, III) are bipolar, recording the electrical difference between two points on the body surface: the left arm–right arm (I), the right arm–left leg (II) and the left leg–left arm (III). These three form the equilateral Einthoven triangle whose apices are the two arms and the left leg. The heart is considered to lie at the centre of this triangle.

The unipolar leads are also recorded from a single limb: VR (right arm), VL (left arm) and VF (left leg). Recording in this manner increases, or augments, the voltage of the unipolar leads and they are, as a consequence, referred to as the augmented limb leads (aVR, aVL, aVF).

The six unipolar chest leads are recorded from the following positions:

V1 Fourth right intercostal space at the sternal border.
V2 Fourth left intercostal space at the sternal border.
V3 Mid-way between V2 and V4.
V4 Fifth left intercostal space in the mid-clavicular line.
V5 Left anterior axillary line at the same horizontal level as V4.
V6 Left mid-axillary line at the same horizontal level as V4 and V5.

The electrical axis

This is a means of summarizing the direction and magnitude of the deflections in the limb leads and indicating the direction of the mean electrical force through the heart. It is derived from these leads and its directions are plotted in relation to the degrees of a circle (Fig. 2.6). Normally it lies between 0° and 110°. Deviations outside these limits,

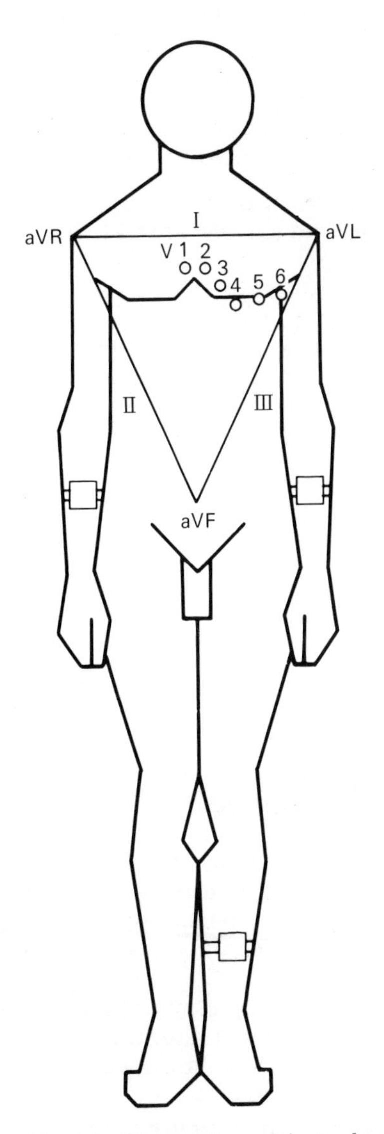

Fig. 2.5 The positions of the twelve ECG leads.

in the directions indicated in Fig. 2.6, constitute left and right axis deviation respectively and signify abnormal patterns of ventricular activation as, for example, in left or right ventricular hypertrophy.

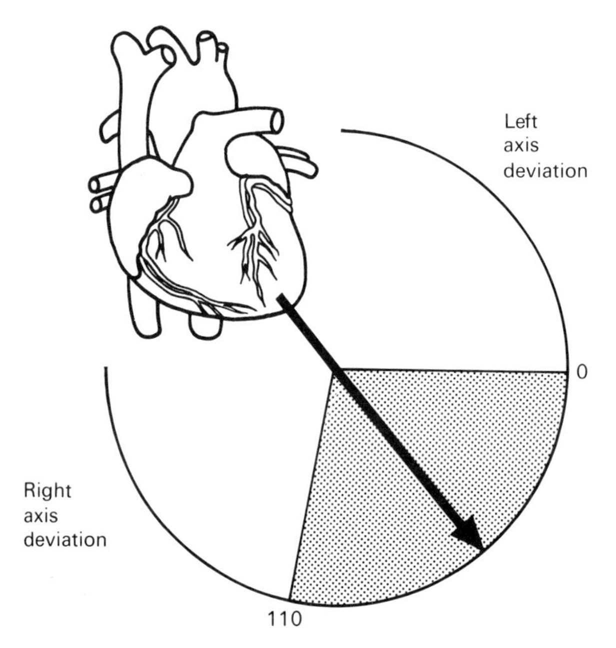

Fig. 2.6 Direction of the electrical axis.

Mechanical events of the cardiac cycle

With electrical stimulation the heart muscle cells contract in sequence, propelling blood forwards and causing a series of pressure changes in the various chambers (Fig. 2.7). Calcium ions are involved in the coupling of the electrical changes to the actual contraction of the myocardial protein fibres. The events are similar on both the right and the left sides of the heart except that the pressures produced in the left ventricle and aorta are some four times greater than those in the right ventricle and pulmonary artery. The following description is for the left side of the heart.

With the onset of ventricular contraction the pressure inside the chamber rises and quickly exceeds that in the atrium, at which point the atrioventricular (mitral) valve closes. The ventricle is now a closed chamber because the aortic valve is also still closed. With continuing contraction the pressure in the ventricles increases very rapidly until it rises above that in the aorta, at which point the aortic valve opens and blood is ejected into the aorta. With the valve open, the pressures in the ventricle and aorta now follow each other for a time but then, as the ventricle relaxes, its pressure falls below that in the aorta, which is sustained by the peripheral resistance, and the aortic valve closes. The ventricle is once again a closed chamber, and remains so until the pressure falls below that in the atrium; then the mitral valve opens and blood flows from the atrium into the ventricle. Much of this flow occurs before atrial contraction as a consequence of the pressure gradient that exists. Atrial contraction subsequently serves as a boost to the filling of the ventricles.

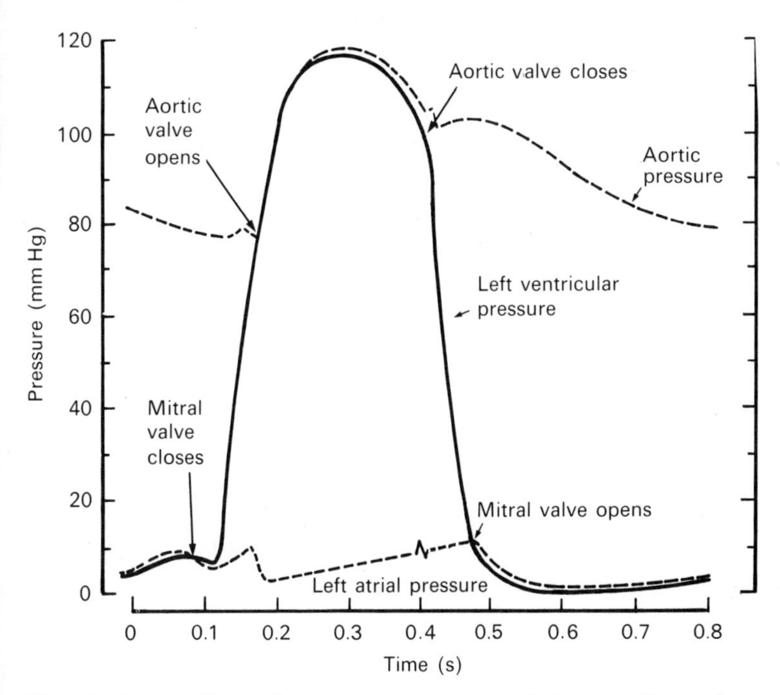

Fig. 2.7 Intracardiac and aortic pressure changes during a cardiac cycle.

Cardiac output

The quantity of blood ejected by the ventricles during a single contraction is termed the stroke volume, and that ejected each minute is the cardiac output, so that cardiac output = stroke volume × heart rate. In a healthy adult at rest the stroke volume varies between 70 and 80 ml. With a heart rate of 70 beats per minute the cardiac output is 4.9–5.6 litres per minute. Values vary with body size and for purposes of comparison are often expressed in relation to body surface area as stroke index (ml/m^2) and cardiac index (litres/m^2).

The mechanisms controlling cardiac output are complex but its magnitude is principally determined by the metabolic activity of the tissues. Any increase is achieved by increasing both the heart rate and the stroke volume. Very high values can be achieved; for instance, during strenuous exercise the output can rise by up to 30 litres per minute or more.

Stroke volume is therefore an expression of the efficiency of the heart pump in dealing with the venous return. Its magnitude is determined by three factors: pre-load, myocardial contractility and after-load.

Pre-load

The more the ventricle fills with blood, the more its muscle is stretched and the greater is the ensuing contraction. This is one way of describing Starling's law of the heart which was originally stated as 'The law of the heart is thus the same as the law of muscular tissue generally that the energy of contraction, however measured, is a function of the length of the muscle fibre'.

Therefore the greater the volume of blood in the ventricles at the end of diastole, the larger will be the stroke volume; there is a well defined relationship between ventricular end-diastolic volume (or pressure) and cardiac output which, when represented graphically, is called a ventricular function curve (Fig. 2.8). The magnitude of the ventricular end-diastolic volume depends on the venous return and the state of the myocardium.

If the atrioventricular valves are normal then the mean atrial pressure is representative of the end-diastolic pressure in the ventricles and is used clinically as a measure of ventricular filling.

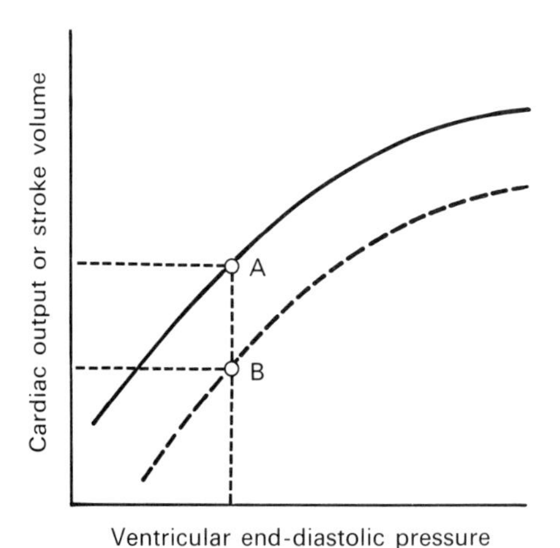

Fig. 2.8 Ventricular function curves: change from curve A to curve B represents a decrease in myocardial contractility.

Myocardial contractility

Myocardial contractility is a difficult characteristic to define. It is a term used to describe the efficiency of muscle contraction for a given degree of stretch. If, for instance, the ventricular end-diastolic volume remains constant, an increase in the myocardial contractility leads to an increase in stroke volume (Fig. 2.8).

It is affected by:

1. the beta sympathetic nervous system, an increased activity of which increases contractility;
2. myocardial depressants such as hypoxia, hypercapnia and acidosis, all of which reduce contractility.

Many of the drugs used in intensive therapy effect contractility (inotropic action) and are often given specifically for this purpose. For example, it is increased by dopamine and isoprenaline, a positive inotropic action and depressed by the beta-blocking drugs and certain anti-dysrhythmics, a negative inotropic action.

After-load

With a given pre-load and level of contractility the stroke volume is further influenced by the degree of shortening of the ventricular muscle fibres that occurs during systole. This, in turn, is related to the resistance to the ejection of blood offered by the systemic and pulmonary circulations, the after-load. The higher the after-load the less able are the muscle cells to shorten during systole, and the stroke volume is lower. The arterial pressure, because of its relation to peripheral resistance, provides an indication of the level of the afterload.

Measurement of the cardiac output

Clinically, the size of the cardiac output is assessed indirectly from the state of the cutaneous and renal circulations, and can be classed as high, normal, or low—approximations that are adequate for a large number of clinical situations. From time to time, however, it is necessary to have an accurate and direct measurement.

A convenient technique, that can be used at the bedside, is the thermodilution method. A known amount of cold saline is injected rapidly into the right atrium and, by contact with the blood flowing through the right side of the heart, its temperature is increased by an amount proportional to the size of the blood flow (cardiac output). The actual temperature change is sensed by a thermistor in the tip of a flotation catheter in the pulmonary artery and, knowing this, the cardiac output can be calculated.

Distribution of the cardiac output

In the resting subject the cardiac output is apportioned to the various regional circulations:

	ml/min		ml/min
Splanchnic	1400	Brain	750
Muscle	1200	Skin	500
Kidneys	1100	Heart	250

Redistribution of the cardiac output, as dictated by the changing metabolic requirements of the various organs, can be effected by local variations in arteriolar resistance—a mechanism that is crucial for maintaining the circulation to certain vital structures when the output falls.

Coronary circulation

Whilst the heart muscle furnishes the driving pressure for the coronary circulation, it also offers a phasic resistance to the blood flow by its contraction around the coronary vessels. The main blood flow therefore occurs during diastole rather than systole and is highly dependent on the level of the aortic diastolic pressure. As the heart rate increases, the duration of diastole becomes relatively less; with very high rates there may be a reduction in coronary flow.

Relationship between blood flow and pressure

The quantity of fluid flowing along any cylindrical tube is directly proportional to the pressure driving it and inversely proportional to the resistance offered by the tube. This is largely determined by the cross-sectional area of the tube and, hence, its radius. A small reduction in the radius produces a relatively large increase in resistance, and vice versa. The pressure/flow relationship can be simply stated as:

$$\text{Flow} = \frac{\text{Pressure}}{\text{Resistance}} \quad \text{or} \quad \text{Pressure} = \text{Flow} \times \text{resistance}$$

This is a most important expression highlighting the fact that two separate variables affect pressure. A normal pressure can therefore exist in association with a reduced flow provided that the resistance increases proportionately, a concept of singular importance for the understanding and management of circulatory failure.

Arterial pressure

Applying the pressure/flow relationship to the circulation it is apparent that the pressure of blood flowing along an artery depends on the magnitude of the flow and the resistance offered to it by the vessel. For the larger arteries this can be stated as:

Mean arterial pressure = Cardiac output × Total peripheral resistance

It applies equally to both the systemic and the pulmonary circulations. Blood flow is the same in each of these but the resistance to flow is much less in the lungs and therefore the pulmonary arterial pressure is only about one-fifth that in the systemic circulation.

Most of the resistance to blood flow occurs in the arterioles and accordingly the main fall in pressure in the circulation is across these vessels.

Changes of arteriolar resistance are effected through variations in the tone of the smooth muscle in their walls. This is normally maintained in a partially contracted (tonic) state by sympathetic nerve activity, variations of which affect vessel diameter. The parasympathetic division plays little part in controlling peripheral resistance.

Control of blood pressure is effected reflexly. Afferent nerve impulses pass from pressure receptors in the walls of the aorta to inhibit the activity of the vasomotor centre in the brain stem. Efferent nerve impulses pass from this centre along the sympathetic nerves to the arterioles. When, for example, blood pressure falls, the number of impulses passing to the vasomotor centre is reduced. Its activity is increased and this is reflected by a greater sympathetic activity, constriction of arterioles, and a rise in peripheral resistance which tends to restore the arterial pressure to its original value.

The tone of arteriolar smooth muscle is also influenced by local changes in its chemical environment; hypoxia and hypercapnia cause vasodilatation.

Central venous pressure (CVP)

Central venous pressure (CVP) is synonymous with right atrial pressure and is a complex phenomenon having a number of determinants (Fig. 2.9). Its value reflects the state of balance between venous return to the heart, venous tone and heart function; variations also occur with changes in intrathoracic pressure and intrapericardial pressure. CVP increases when venous return and venous tone increase or when cardiac function deteriorates, and vice versa.

Because it is the resultant of a number of variables, interpretation of a single measurement is difficult should more than one of them change. For instance, if impaired cardiac function coexists with a low venous return, the CVP may be within normal limits. Similarly, a rise in venous tone can offset the effect of a reduction in venous return.

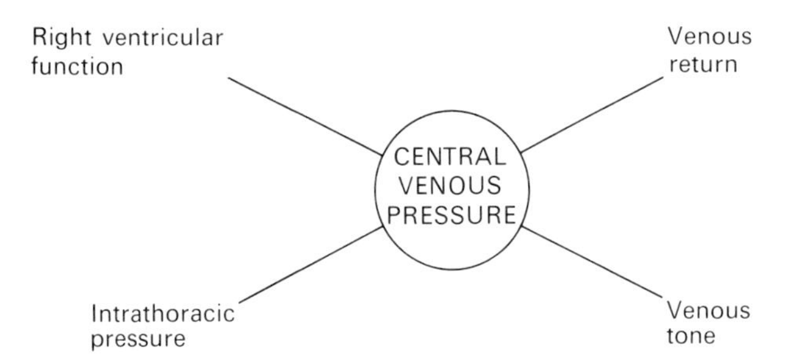

Fig. 2.9 Determinants of central venous pressure.

Measurement

A radio-opaque catheter is passed into the right atrium from an antecubital, subclavian or internal jugular vein. The femoral veins are unsuitable because of the high risk of sepsis.

After insertion, its position must be checked on a portable chest x-ray because not infrequently catheters double back on themselves, pass into the veins of the neck or enter the right ventricle. With the catheter in a suitable position, the CVP can be measured intermittently using a simple fluid manometer containing dextrose or saline, or continuously with a transducer.

A fluid manometer is a branch of a giving set, linked to the venous catheter via a three-way tap, and mounted on a centimetre scale (Fig. 2.10).

Normal values

Measured from the mid-axillary line the normal range of CVP is 5–10 cm H_2O (0.5–1.0 kPa); from the sternal angle it is 0–5 cmH_2O (0–0.5 kPa). For a transducer the units are millimetres of mercury (mm Hg) and the normal range is 3–8 (or 0.4–1.1 kPa).

Intermittent positive pressure ventilation (IPPV) increases the mean intrathoracic pressure by up to 5 mm Hg, (0.7 kPa) which is reflected by a rise in CVP. This must be taken into account when interpreting the CVP of ventilated patients.

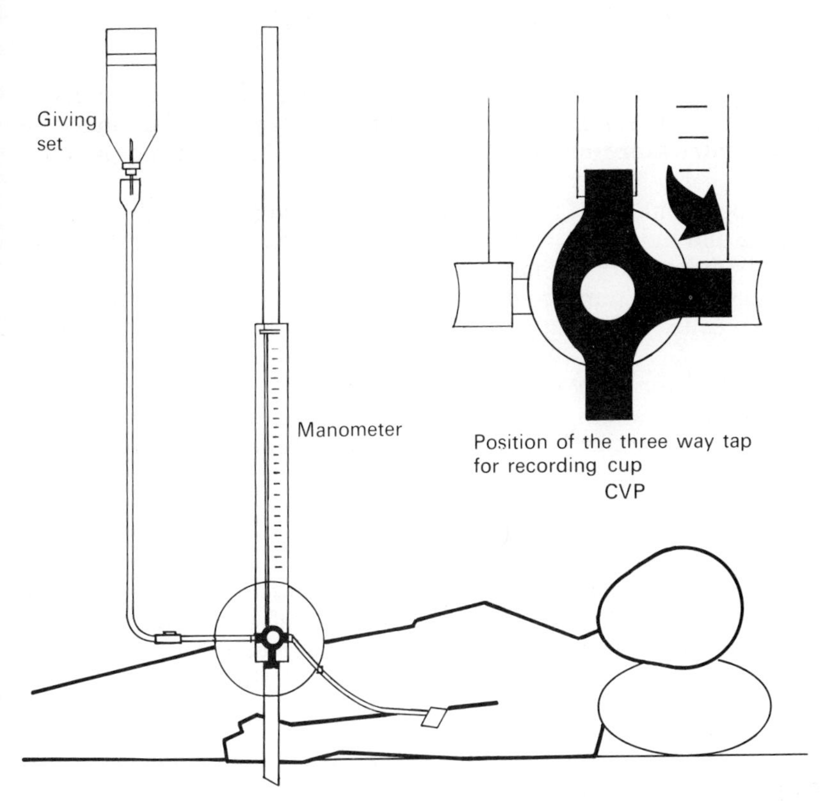

Fig. 2.10 A fluid manometer system for measuring CVP.

Clinical application

From theoretical considerations it would appear that the CVP might be used to assess blood volume (equated with venous return), right ventricular function and, by inference from this, left ventricular function. In certain situations it can be an extremely helpful measurement but equally it has important limitations which are not always appreciated.

Blood volume
In pure hypovolaemia the CVP is a reliable indicator for assessing the extent of the blood volume depletion, monitoring fluid replacement and preventing over-transfusion; serial measurements are particularly helpful.

In those patients where recurrent fluid losses may arise, such as re-bleeding from a peptic ulcer, CVP is a sensitive monitor. It often falls before changes appear in pulse rate or blood pressure.

Right ventricular function

If the tricuspid valve is normal, the CVP equals the end-diastolic pressure in the right ventricle and, as such, it is an index of right ventricular function. When the function is impaired the CVP rises.

The performance of the right ventricle is affected directly by heart disease and indirectly by disturbances in the pulmonary circulation such as pulmonary embolism.

In pericardial tamponade, interference with right ventricular filling can cause a sudden and steep rise in CVP.

Left ventricular function

Left atrial pressure is an index of left ventricular function in the same way that the CVP relates to right ventricular function. A knowledge of left rather than right ventricular function is often far more important in many acute circulatory disorders such as cardiogenic shock or pulmonary oedema. In such conditions the level of left atrial pressure is deduced from the CVP. Normally there is a relationship between the two but in many diseased states this no longer holds and then using CVP to estimate left ventricular function becomes very unreliable and can lead to serious errors of management. Patients with severe left ventricular failure and pulmonary oedema can have a normal CVP.

Pulmonary wedge pressure (PWP)

The deficiencies mentioned above in CVP can be overcome by measurement of the pulmonary 'wedge' pressure (PWP), which is identical to the left atrial pressure and so provides a direct estimate of left ventricular function.

The measurement is made using a flotation or Swan–Ganz catheter which has a small inflatable balloon at its tip (Fig. 2.11). It is attached to a transducer and is usually inserted from an antecubital or subclavian vein. When the tip reaches the region of the superior vena cava, the balloon is inflated with either air or carbon dioxide; this facilitates its passage through the right atrium and ventricle to the pulmonary artery where it eventually wedges in a small peripheral branch and records a 'wedge pressure'. X-ray screening during the procedure is not necessary; the location of the catheter can be recognized from the pressure waveform recorded by the transducer. Wedging produces a characteristic change in the pulmonary artery pressure trace (Fig. 2.12).

Between measurements, the balloon is deflated and the catheter remains in the main pulmonary artery. Used in this way it can be left *in situ* for up to three days without complications.

The normal PWP ranges from 4 to 12 mmHg (0.5 to 1.6. kPa).

Flotation catheters are now being used much more frequently and PWP is replacing CVP as a measure of cardiac function in many critically ill patients.

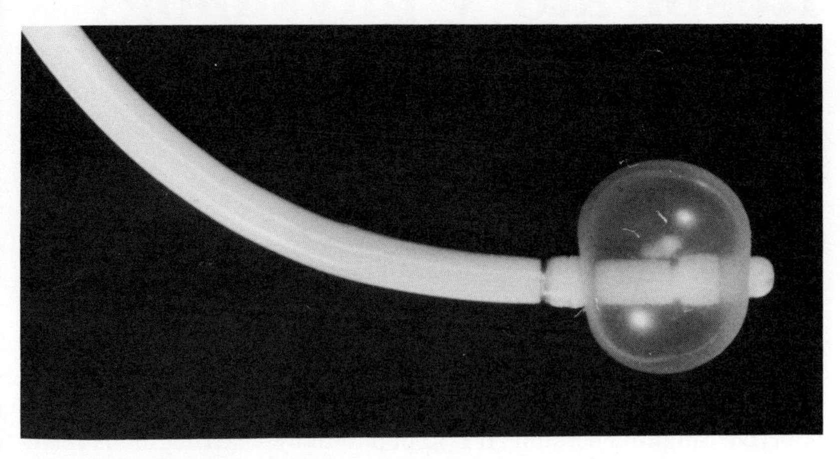

Fig. 2.11 The balloon of a flotation catheter.

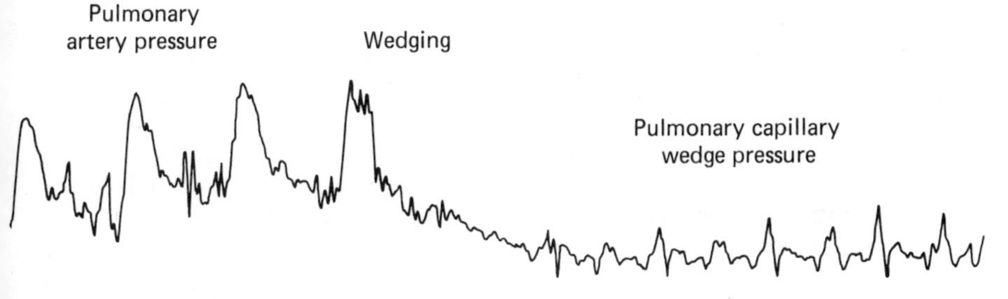

Fig. 2.12 A 'wedge' pressure tracing.

3

Respiratory physiology

Anatomy

The features of particular note are shown in (Fig. 3.1).

The larynx is concerned in the production of the voice and also functions as a sphincteric valve at the entrance to the trachea, preventing food from entering the lower respiratory tract and making effective coughing possible. It is kept patent by a cartilaginous skeleton, and identification of the structures around its opening (Fig. 3.2) is essential for successful tracheal intubation. The position of the vocal cords and the arytenoid cartilages makes them particularly vulnerable to damage from an endotracheal tube.

The trachea continues from the lower border of the larynx. It is a fibromuscular tube about 10–12 cm long and 1.3–2.5 cm wide; its wall is strengthened by U-shaped cartilaginous rings. In the neck the second, third and fourth cartilaginous rings are covered anteriorly by the isthmus of the thyroid gland. Posteriorly it is related to the oesophagus which separates it from the vertebral column.

At the level of the sternal angle it divides into the right and left main bronchi, the point of division is called the carina. The right main bronchus is wider and more directly in line with the trachea than the left, so inhaled foreign bodies and displaced endotracheal tubes tend to pass into it more readily. The main bronchi subdivide many times into smaller and smaller bronchioles which terminate as alveolar ducts leading to alveolar sacs, from which the alveoli arise.

The trachea and larger bronchi are lined by ciliated epithelium and mucus-secreting cells. The movements of the cilia move the mucous layer, by mechanical agitation, in an upward direction. Smooth muscle is present in the walls of the airways as far as the bronchioles. It is supplied by beta 2 sympathetic nerves which relax its tone, dilating the airways—the reason for the cautious use of beta-blocking drugs in patients with asthma.

The lungs are divided into lobes, three on the right and two on the left; each lobe is further subdivided into bronchopulmonary segments with their own segmental bronchus. Each lung is invested by two

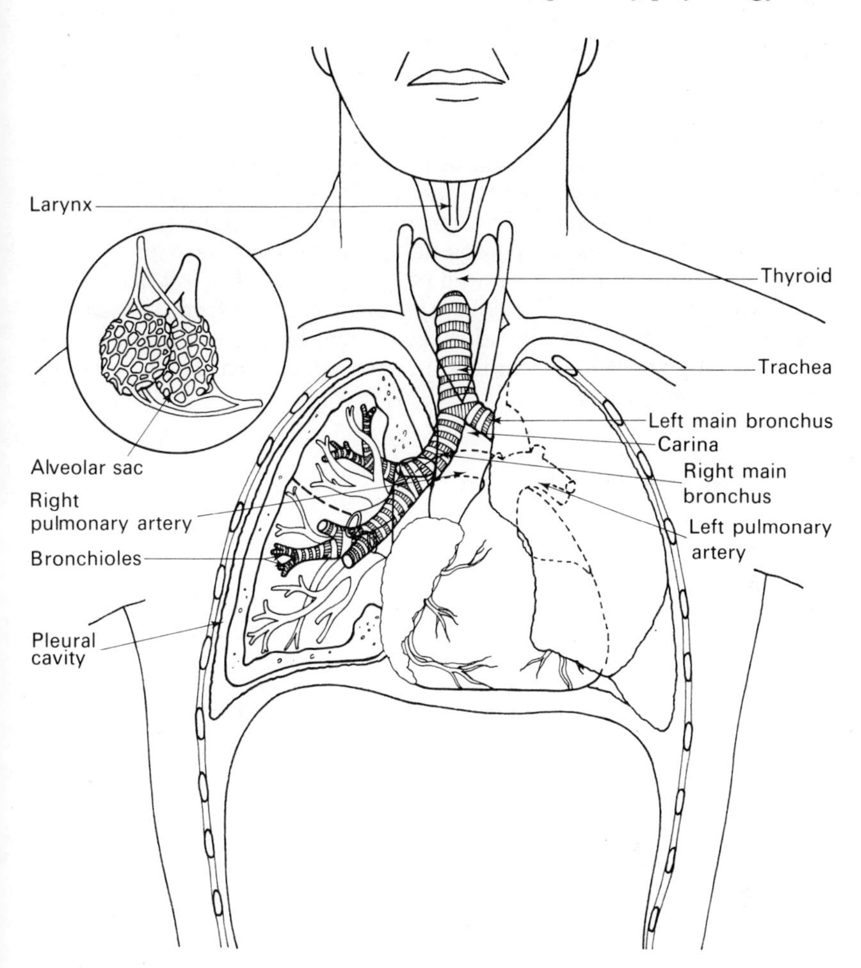

Fig. 3.1 Anatomical features of the respiratory system.

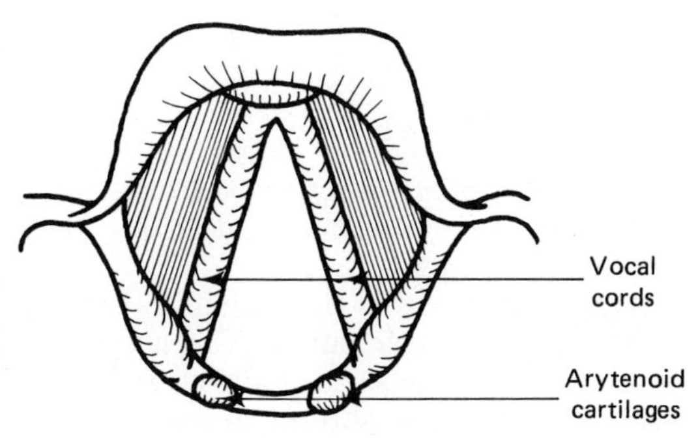

Fig. 3.2 The laryngeal opening.

layers of pleura, visceral and parietal (analogous to the pericardium), separated by a potential space, the pleural cavity (see Fig. 3.1). The pleura has an important role in respiratory movements.

The pulmonary artery arises from the right ventricle and divides into right and left main branches. These subdivide further, giving branches that accompany the branches of the bronchial tree; they end in the alveolar capillaries. The ligamentum arteriosum, the remnant of the ductus arteriosus, passes between the left main pulmonary artery and the aorta. Oxygenated blood returns to the left atrium via four pulmonary veins. The bronchial arteries stem from the ascending aorta. They provide a blood supply for the bronchi and lung tissue, and normally there is no connection between them and the vessels of the pulmonary circulation.

Respiratory or alveolar unit

This term refers to the structures involved in gas exchange: the alveoli and their capillary blood supply.

There are approximately 300 million alveoli in the lungs. Their walls consist of a single layer of cells, called pneumocytes, coated with a film of a lipoprotein, known as surfactant. The origin of surfactant is uncertain but it is necessary for the 'stability' of the alveoli which would otherwise tend to collapse. Loss of surfactant occurs in various forms of the 'respiratory distress syndrome'. The capillaries are lined by endothelial cells resting on a basement membrane. Between the alveolar walls and the capillary network is the interstitial space; lymphatic channels arise from this.

Gas exchange can only take place in alveoli that are both ventilated and have a capillary circulation. For optimal exchange the two components, ventilation (V) and perfusion (Q), must be correctly matched.

The mediastinum is the space between the lungs. It contains the pericardium, the oesophagus, the great vessels, and the vagus, sympathetic and phrenic nerves.

Muscles of respiration

These are the diaphragm and the intercostal muscles. In deep and forced inspiration additional (accessory) muscles are called into play; for example, the pectorals and sternomastoids.

The diaphragm separates the thoracic from the abdominal cavity and arises from the margins of the thoracic outlet. The aorta, the oesophagus and the inferior vena cava pass through it. Its nerve supply, both motor and sensory, is from the phrenic nerve (C3, 4, 5) whose long course from the neck follows the embryological migration of the diaphragm from the cervical region. The height of the diaphragm in the chest varies constantly during respiration and also with the degree of distension of the stomach and the size of the liver.

The intercostal muscles pass between the ribs and are supplied by the intercostal nerves.

During inspiration the movements of the chest wall and diaphragm result in an increase in all diameters of the thorax. This, in turn, produces a negative intrapleural pressure and expansion of the lungs. Conversely, in expiration the muscles relax and the elastic recoil of the lungs reduces their capacity and air is expelled; the intrapleural pressure becomes positive. Inspiration is an active process requiring muscular work expiration is normally passive.

Lung volumes

Normal or tidal breathing occurs in the mid-range of the total lung volume (Fig. 3.3), and the volume of air left in the lungs after normal expiration is termed the functional residual capacity (FRC). Greater excursions of breathing encroach upon the FRC but even at the end of a maximal expiration there is always a residual volume. After expanding the lungs with a maximal inspiration, the volume of the subsequent maximal expiration is called the vital capacity.

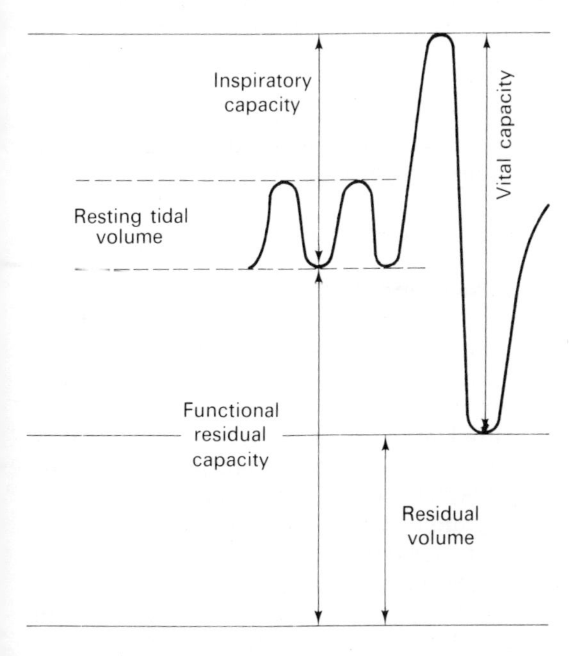

Fig. 3.3 The lung volumes.

Compliance

When a certain volume of air enters the lungs there is an increase in the pressure within them. The less elastic or stiffer the lungs, the greater will be this rise in pressure. A measure of the degree of lung stiffness is called the compliance; the stiffer the lungs, the smaller is the compliance.

Airway resistance

Air flowing into the lungs encounters resistance from the trachea and bronchi (airway resistance), the magnitude of which is proportional to their cross-sectional area. The narrower they are, the higher is the resistance to airflow; in cases of severe asthma, for example, it becomes very high.

Humidification of the inspired air

Humidity is invisible moisture. Two terms are used to describe the humidity of a gas.

Relative humidity refers to the amount of water vapour present in a gas at any temperature, expressed as a percentage of the amount of water vapour which the gas would hold if it were fully saturated at that temperature.

Absolute humidity is a measure of the actual quantity of water vapour present in a unit volume of dry gas at standard temperature and pressure. It is usually expressed in milligrams of water/litre.

Increasing the temperature of a gas increases the amount of water vapour it can hold.

Inspired air acquires both heat and moisture during its passage through the respiratory tract. The greatest contribution comes from the nasal and oropharynx, and when the air reaches the upper trachea it has a relative humidity close to 100 per cent (44 mg water/litre) and a temperature somewhere between 32 and 36°C. In the alveoli it is fully saturated at a temperature of 37°C. Under normal conditions there is a loss of 250 ml of water and 350 calories per day from the respiratory tract. Gases with temperatures greater than 40°C cause hyperthermia and laryngeal spasm, whilst temperatures below 30°C depress ciliary activity.

Dry gases are harmful to the respiratory tract and cause drying of the bronchial secretions. When the pharynx is bypassed by either an endotracheal tube or a tracheostomy, it is essential to humidify the inspired gases artificially.

Radiology of the lungs (Fig. 3.4)

The trachea can normally be seen as a central dark (air-containing) shadow overlying the spinous processes of the upper thoracic vertebrae. The point of bifurcation into the two main bronchi, the carina, is an important reference point for checking the position of the tips of endotracheal and tracheostomy tubes.

The lungs appear as dark areas on each side of the mediastinal shadow; each is crossed by a fine pattern of lines radiating from the hila—these represent the small pulmonary vessels. Below are the shadows of the diaphragm, the right dome normally being 1–3 cm higher than the left because of the underlying liver.

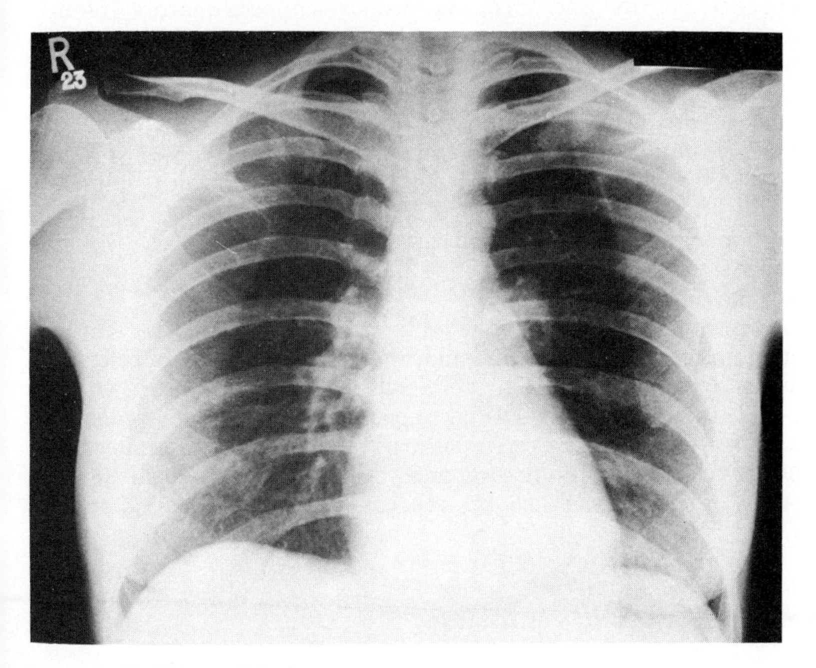

Fig. 3.4 Radiology of the lungs.

Function of the lungs

The essential function of the lungs is to add oxygen to, and remove carbon dioxide from, the pulmonary capillary blood. This involves three processes: pulmonary ventilation, exchange of oxygen and carbon dioxide in the alveolar units, and transport of these gases by the blood.

Pulmonary ventilation

This replenishes the oxygen in the alveoli and removes the carbon dioxide produced by the body. It is described in terms of the volume of air that passes into, or out of, the lungs—the tidal volume being an expression of ventilation per breath. This multiplied by the number of breaths per minute gives the minute ventilation or minute volume. With a tidal volume of 500 ml and a respiratory rate of 15 per minute the minute volume equals 15 × 500, or 7.5 litres per minute.

Only part of a tidal volume, two-thirds in a healthy subject, actually ventilates the alveoli. The remainder fills the upper respiratory tract, trachea and bronchi, where no gas exchange occurs. This is the 'dead space' volume and normally measures approximately 150 ml. This value may be reduced by as much as 50 per cent with a tracheostomy and by 30 per cent with an endotracheal tube. If a patient is being artificially ventilated, the ventilator tubing provides a mechanical dead space. The effective or alveolar minute ventilation is therefore equal to the tidal volume minus the dead space volume, multiplied by the respiratory rate per minute. It is normally adjusted to maintain the alveolar level of carbon dioxide constant and is consequently matched to the carbon dioxide production of the body. The best indication of ventilatory efficiency is therefore the arterial carbon dioxide tension (P_{CO_2}).

Control of ventilation is effected by the respiratory centre in the brain stem which receives information from the brain, muscles and tissues via nerves, and from the blood by chemical stimuli. On the basis of this it adjusts its activity to produce the appropriate level of ventilation. The efferent impulses are transmitted to the muscles of respiration via the spinal cord and the related peripheral nerves. Integrity of this neuromuscular axis is essential for normal ventilation.

Chemical control of ventilation

The most important factor in the rhythmic pattern of breathing is the carbon dioxide tension (P_{CO_2}) of the blood affecting chemoreceptors, in the medulla, that are linked to the respiratory centre. An increase in the P_{CO_2} of the blood increases both the rate and depth of breathing. A reduction, induced by voluntary hyperventilation, results in a period of reduced ventilation or even temporary apnoea.

The respiratory centre is also directly affected by changes in blood pH, a fall in pH increasing ventilation and a rise reducing it.

Ventilation is less sensitive to changes of blood oxygen tension (P_{O_2}). The usual effect of hypoxia is to increase the rate and depth of breathing through action on the peripheral chemoreceptors in the carotid and aortic bodies. In many clinical conditions hypoxia and acidosis are associated, and it remains a matter for debate as to which is the dominant stimulus to ventilation.

Exchange of oxygen and carbon dioxide in the alveolar units

Air contains 21 per cent oxygen and 0.04 per cent of carbon dioxide; the remainder consists of nitrogen plus water vapour. Air in the alveoli contains 14 per cent oxygen, 6 per cent carbon dioxide and is saturated with water vapour at body temperature. Each of the gases contributes to the total pressure in proportion to its concentration; this principle is stated formally in Dalton's law of partial pressures.

Atmospheric pressure at sea level is 760 mm Hg (101.3 kPa); since oxygen forms 21 per cent of the total, its partial pressure is 21 per cent of 760, that is 160 mm Hg (21.2 kPa). In the alveoli the water vapour has a partial pressure of 47 mm Hg (6.3 kPa); the total pressure of the other gases is therefore (760 − 47) mmHg, that is 713 mmHg (95 kPa). The partial pressure of oxygen in the alveoli is therefore 14 per cent of 713, approximately 100 mmHg (13.3 kPa); that of carbon dioxide is 40 mmHg (5.3 kPa).

In the alveoli, oxygen passes into, and carbon dioxide out of, the blood by diffusion because of the pressure gradients that exist; the partial pressure of oxygen in blood returning to the lungs is approximately 40 mmHg (5.3 kPa) and that of carbon dioxide 46 mmHg (6.1 kPa). After the blood has traversed the pulmonary capillaries these pressures have equilibrated with those in the alveoli and the partial pressure of oxygen in arterial blood ($P\text{O}_2$) is between 95 and 100 mmHg (12.7 and 13.3 kPa) and that of carbon dioxide ($P\text{CO}_2$) is 40 mmHg (5.3 kPa).

The passage of oxygen and carbon dioxide between alveolar gas and capillary blood is, as already stated, a process of diffusion and no active secretory mechanisms are involved.

If such exchange is to occur, then of course the alveoli must be ventilated with air and also perfused by capillary blood. In an ideal lung, inspiration would draw air of the same composition into each separate alveolus and the pulmonary blood flow would be distributed equally to all the alveolar capillaries. In reality this ideal is never attained and in disease states the relationship can be grossly disturbed.

Ventilation/perfusion (V/Q) ratio

The matching of ventilation (V) and perfusion (Q) in health results in an arterial $P\text{O}_2$ of 100 mmHg (13.3 kPa) and a $P\text{CO}_2$ of 40 mmHg (5.3

kPa). In abnormal situations the relationship, expressed as the V/Q ratio, may be altered in two ways.

Ventilation may be reduced to alveoli that are normally perfused; V is low and Q is normal, hence the V/Q ration is reduced. This imbalance results in a difference of oxygen tension between the alveolar gas (A) and the arterial blood (a), the so-called alveolar–capillary or (A–a) gradient. The size of the gradient is an index of its severity.

On the other hand, perfusion may fall to a greater extent than ventilation and the V/Q ratio increases. This effectively increases the dead space volume, resulting in a fall in alveolar oxygen and a rise in carbon dioxide.

The hypoxia of respiratory failure arises almost totally from V/Q abnormalities. Impairment of diffusion, once thought to be a contributory factor, is rarely significant in acute disease.

Transport of oxygen in the blood

Oxygen is transported in two ways.

1. *In simple solution, the oxygen being physically dissolved in the plasma.* This quantity is proportional to its partial pressure, and at 100 mmHg (13.3 kPa) 0.3 ml of oxygen is dissolved in every 100 ml of blood. This is a relatively small volume but the partial pressure of the gas in solution is very important in determining the quantity of oxygen that is transferred from the blood to the tissues.

In combination with haemoglobin in the red cells. One gram of haemoglobin combines with 1.34 ml of oxygen. Normally there are 14 g of haemoglobin per 100 ml of blood so that nearly 19 ml of oxygen is carried in this way in each 100 ml of blood. Because of the chemical structure of haemoglobin, the combination between it and oxygen to form oxyhaemoglobin is not a linear process but follows a course that is described by a sigmoid, or S-shaped, curve (Fig. 3.5).

This shape has great practical significance. From Fig. 3.5 it can be seen that with pressures of oxygen in excess of 60 mmHg (8 kPa), because the curve is flat, only small amounts of oxygen combine with haemoglobin for relatively large increases in pressure. For this reason there is little point, when treating patients with acute respiratory failure, in striving to achieve arterial oxygen tensions much greater than 60 mmHg (8 kPa). Below the 60 mmHg point, however, the situation is quite different and between 40 and 60 mmHg (5.3 and 8 kPa) the curve has a steep slope so that much greater quantities of oxygen react for smaller changes in pressure. Increasing a patient's PO_2 anywhere along this section of the curve produces a relatively large increase in the oxygen content.

It is also important to appreciate that the dissociation curve does not have a fixed position but can shift, to the right or left, in response to certain chemical changes in the blood (Fig. 3.5). For instance, with a fall in the blood pH (acidosis) the curve moves to the right; with a rise in pH (alkalosis) it moves to the left. Also, an increase in carbon dioxide tension shifts the curve to the right and a decrease to the left. A right shift means that the haemoglobin has less affinity for oxygen and releases it more readily. Conversely, with a left shift the haemoglobin has a greater affinity for oxygen.

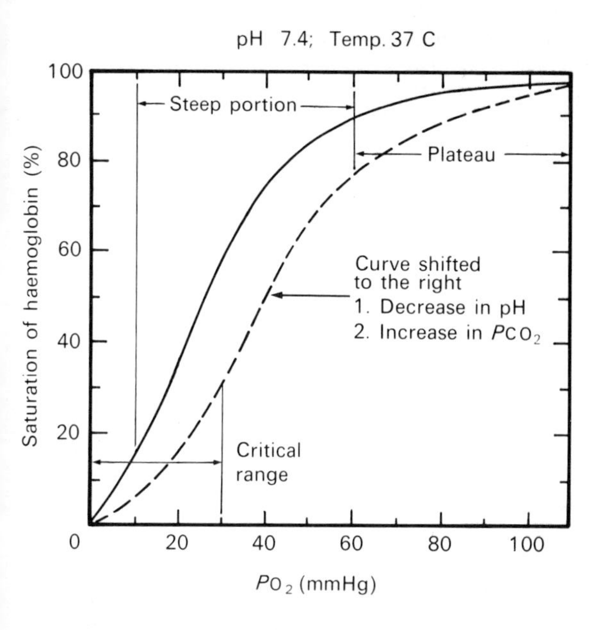

Fig. 3.5 The oxyhaemoglobin dissociation curve.

Transfer of oxygen from blood to tissues

The transfer of oxygen from the capillaries to the tissue cells is governed entirely by diffusion. The tissue oxygen tension is around 40 mmHg (5.3 kPa) and oxygen will diffuse from the blood, where the P_{O_2} is 100 mmHg (13.3 kPa), until there is an equalization of pressures. The quantity of oxygen released depends on its dissociation from haemoglobin which is faciliated by the low tissue pH and high P_{CO_2} both of which move the dissociation curve to the right. The situation is reversed in the lungs and the curve moves to the left increasing the affinity of haemoglobin for oxygen.

In summary, the total quantity of oxygen that is supplied to the tissues depends upon three factors.

1. The arterial oxygen tension.
2. The haemoglobin content of the blood.
3. The cardiac output.

Transport of carbon dioxide in the blood

Carbon dioxide is carried in the blood from the tissues to the lungs in three ways.

1. *In solution*. Carbon dioxide is more soluble than oxygen and the amount in solution is proportional to the pressure.
2. *Combined with blood proteins*: especially haemoglobin in the form of carbamino compounds.
3. *In the form of bicarbonate*. This constitutes the largest part. It is transported as sodium bicarbonate in the plasma and potassium bicarbonate in the red cells according to the equation.

$$\underset{\text{carbon dioxide}}{CO_2} + \underset{\text{water}}{H_2O} \rightleftharpoons \underset{\text{carbonic acid}}{H_2CO_3} \rightleftharpoons \underset{\text{hydrogen ion}}{H^+} + \underset{\text{bicarbonate}}{HCO_3^-}$$

The reaction between water and carbon dioxide to form carbonic acid is catalysed by the enzyme carbonic anhydrase which is present in high concentrations in the red cells. The carbonic acid dissociates into hydrogen ions and bicarbonate, the hydrogen ions are buffered by haemoglobin and the bicarbonate combines with potassium and sodium ions. In the blood leaving the tissue the reaction is towards hydrogen ions and bicarbonate but at the lungs it is reversed with the liberation of carbon dioxide.

Elimination of carbon dioxide

In the lungs the alveolar tension of carbon dioxide is lower than the P_{CO_2} of mixed venous blood flowing into the pulmonary capillaries. It therefore diffuses out into the alveoli and is 'washed away' by ventilation.

Test of respiratory function

There are many different tests that might be employed to assess the varied aspects of respiration. In an ITU only a few simple tests, that can be carried out easily at the patient's bedside, are needed.

The tidal volume, minute volume and vital capacity can all be measured using a Wright respirometer (Fig. 3.6). In this the movement of air produced by the breath causes a two-bladed rotor to revolve. The rotations are recorded, by means of internal gears, as volumes of gas on a dial similar to that used in a watch with minute and second hands; one full sweep of the large hand corresponds to a volume of 100 litres. The meter only responds to gas flow in one direction. An electronic version of the respirometer is also available with a meter display and electrical outlets for a recorder; the move-

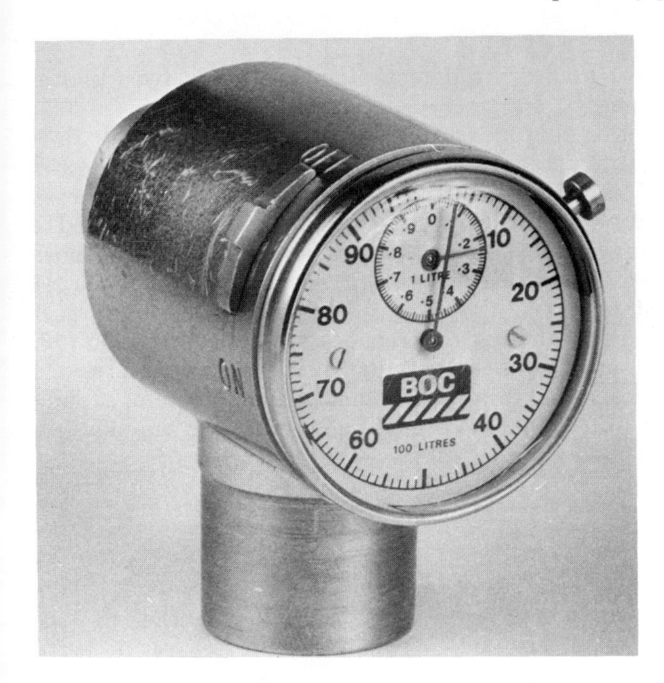

Fig. 3.6 A Wright respirometer.

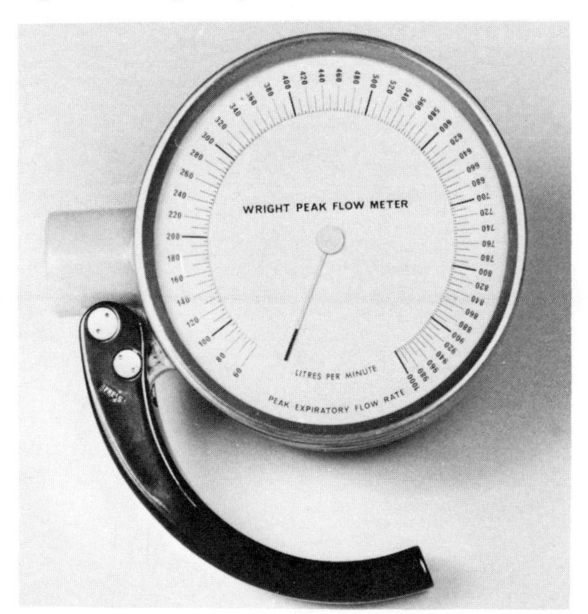

Fig. 3.7 A Wright peak flow meter.

ments of the rotor blades are detected automatically by a photo-electric mechanism.

The peak flow rate is a measure of the maximal rate of air flow achieved during a forced expiration. The patient inspires fully and then 'blows out' as fast as possible through the mouthpiece of a Wright peak flow meter (Fig. 3.7). This consists of a vane connected to a moving recording needle; the more forceful the expiration, the more will the needle travel around the dial which is calibrated in litres per minute. The instrument is light and relatively small in size.

The peak flow rate falls with increasing airway obstruction and provides a good measurement for documenting the progress of asthmatic patients. A healthy person should have a rate of around 600 litres per minute, whereas a moderate asthmatic may show a value of only 200 litres per minute.

4

Body fluids and the kidneys

Terminology

Electrolytes

These acquire their name because in solution they are dissociated into ions and can conduct an electric current. For example, sodium chloride (NaCl) in solution dissociates into sodium ions (Na) and chloride ions (Cl); the sodium ion carries a positive electric charge (Na^+) and the chloride a negative one (Cl^-). Positively charged ions such as sodium, potassium and calcium are referred to as cations because they move towards the cathode when an electric current is passed. In the same way, negatively charged ions such as chloride and bicarbonate are referred to as anions because they move towards the anode. In a solution the number of cations must balance the number of anions.

Osmolality

Dissolved solutes diminish the tendency of water to escape across a membrane into another solution. The extent to which solutes do this depends chiefly upon the total number of dissolved particles per unit weight of solvent rather than the chemical nature of the particles.

The total molar concentration of particles *per kilogram* of solvent is called the osmolality; for plasma the normal range is 275–295 mmol/kg.

Osmolarity

The molar concentration of dissolved particles *per litre* of solvent is also used and, for biological solutions, has the same value as osmolality because a litre of solution contains close to 1 kg of water.

Osmotic pressure

The distribution of water between two solutions that are separated by a membrane, which is impermeable to all solutes, is determined by the osmolality of the two solutions. Water will diffuse across the membrane from the low to the high osmolality solution until the osmolality is equal on both sides of the membrane. The pressure that would need to be applied to prevent this movement is the osmotic pressure of the solution. Therefore the higher the osmolality of a solution, the greater is the osmotic pressure it exerts.

In the body the capillary membrane is permeable to all but very large molecules, such as the blood proteins, and therefore it is these that are responsible for the effective osmotic pressure of the plasma when compared to the interstitial fluid. The total osmotic pressure of plasma is equivalent to about 7 atmospheres and the proportion of this due to plasma proteins in only some 25 mmHg (3.3 kPa). Nevertheless, this proportion is of great physiological importance since it determines the distribution of fluid between blood and interstitial fluid.

The body fluids

These consist of water containing crystalloids and colloids. In health their volume and composition remains remarkably constant in spite of many influences for change. It is to Claude Bernard that we owe the concept of the constancy of the internal environment, the *milieu interieur*, that is essential for normal cell function.

Distribution

The total volume of body water comprises between 50 and 70 per cent of the body weight. The proportion is related to the mass of the lean tissues rather than to the total body weight so that, for instance, in an obese person it is much lower.

Body water resides in two major compartments (Fig. 4.1): inside the cells as intracellular fluid (ICF), 30–35 per cent of body weight; and outside them as extracellular fluid (ECF), 15–20 per cent of body weight. The ECF consists of the blood plasma, 3–5 per cent of body weight, the interstitial fluid, the lymph and the fluid in serous cavities.

Each of these volumes, the ICF and the ECF, is a complex solution and whilst it is convenient to separate them into compartments it must be realized that they are functionally integrated.

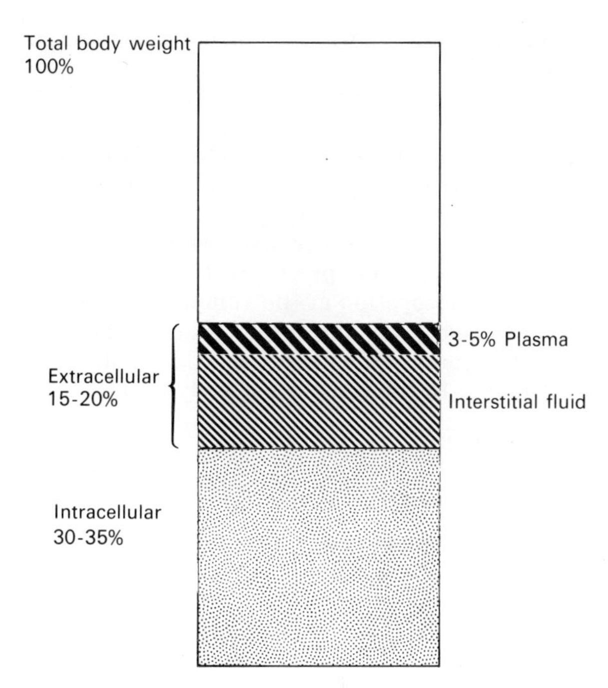

Fig. 4.1 Division of the body fluids.

Composition

ECF differs markedly from ICF in its chemical composition. It contains relatively large amounts of sodium and small amounts of potassium. In contrast, the ICF has high concentrations of potassium and magnesium and a low concentration of sodium. The difference is maintained by an active energy-consuming mechanism in the cell membranes, the so-called 'sodium-pump'. Cell membranes are permeable to water, so the ECF and ICF have equal osmolalities.

Plasma and interstitial fluid are continuous with respect to their electrolyte composition, but the capillaries are not normally permeable to protein molecules which remain in the plasma and are responsible for the important differences of osmotic pressure between the two fluids.

Exchange of fluid across the capillaries

Blood at the arterial end of the capillaries exerts a hydrostatic pressure of approximately 32 mmHg (4.3 kPa). This falls progressively along the length of the capillary and at the venous end is around 12 mmHg (Fig. 4.2). Because capillaries are permeable to all constituents of plasma, except proteins, there is an osmotic force of 25 mmHg (3.3 kPa), due to the proteins (mainly albumin), tending to hold fluid in the capillaries. Consequently, at the arterial end of each capillary there are two opposing forces: the blood pressure, forcing fluid out, and the osmotic pressure of the plasma proteins, holding it in. Since the hydrostatic pressure is greater by 7 mmHg (0.9 kPa), fluid flows out of the capillaries into the tissue spaces. At the venous end the osmotic pressure now exceeds the hydrostatic pressure and fluid returns to the circulation. This process of filtration at the arterial end of a capillary and absorption at the venous end goes on continually in all capillary networks; the mechanisms were first described by Starling in 1896. Some of the interstitial fluid is drained away by lymphatics, returning to the circulation as lymph.

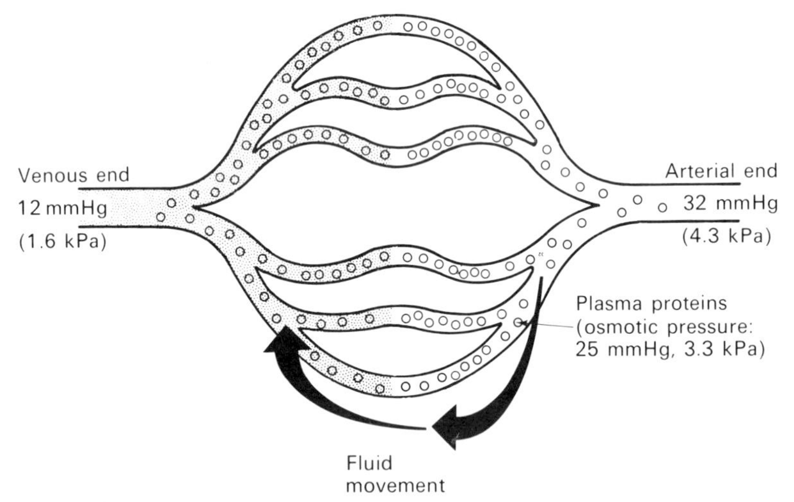

Fig. 4.2 Fluid exchange across the capillaries.

The regulation of the circulating blood volume is largely dependent upon the balance between fluid in the vessels and in the tissue spaces, as governed by these mechanisms. An excess of interstitial fluid (oedema) at the expense of the circulating volume can occur if there is a fall in the plasma albumin, a rise in the pressure at the venous end of the capillary or an increase in the permeability of the capillary wall that allows protein to leak out. All of these have important clinical associations.

The kidneys: anatomy

The kidneys are situated retroperitoneally on either side of the vertebral column (T12–L3). In the centre of the medial border of each kidney is the hilum through which the renal artery enters and the renal vein and ureter leave.

Two main renal arteries, a right and a left, arise from the abdominal aorta. They divide into numerous branches from which the afferent arterioles of the glomeruli arise. The renal veins drain into the inferior vena cava.

Renal blood flow amounts to just over 1 litre per minute, one-fifth of the total cardiac output. This is a very large blood flow relative to the size of the kidneys and reflects the dominance of their excretory role.

The nephron (Fig. 4.3)

The functional unit of the kidney is the nephron and each kidney contains approximately one million. A single nephron is a tubular structure, one end of which is closed and invaginated by a cluster of capillaries to form the glomerulus and the other end drains into the collecting ducts. It is possible to lose up to three-quarters of the nephrons without ill effect because the remaining nephrons compensate.

The glomerulus

The glomeruli lie in the cortex of the kidney, each consisting of a network of capillaries surrounded by the expanded closed end of the nephron. Blood enters the glomerular capillaries from a short afferent arteriole and leaves them by an efferent arteriole. The anatomical arrangement of the glomeruli provides a large surface area for the filtration of the blood.

The renal tubule

This is the continuation of the nephron from the glomerulus. Each tubule has a long and tortuous course through the kidney substance and finally drains into the pelvis of the ureter. A single tubule is subdivided into three sections: the proximal tubule continuing from the glomerulus, the loop of Henle in the renal medulla and the distal tubule which is again situated in the cortex (Fig. 4.3).

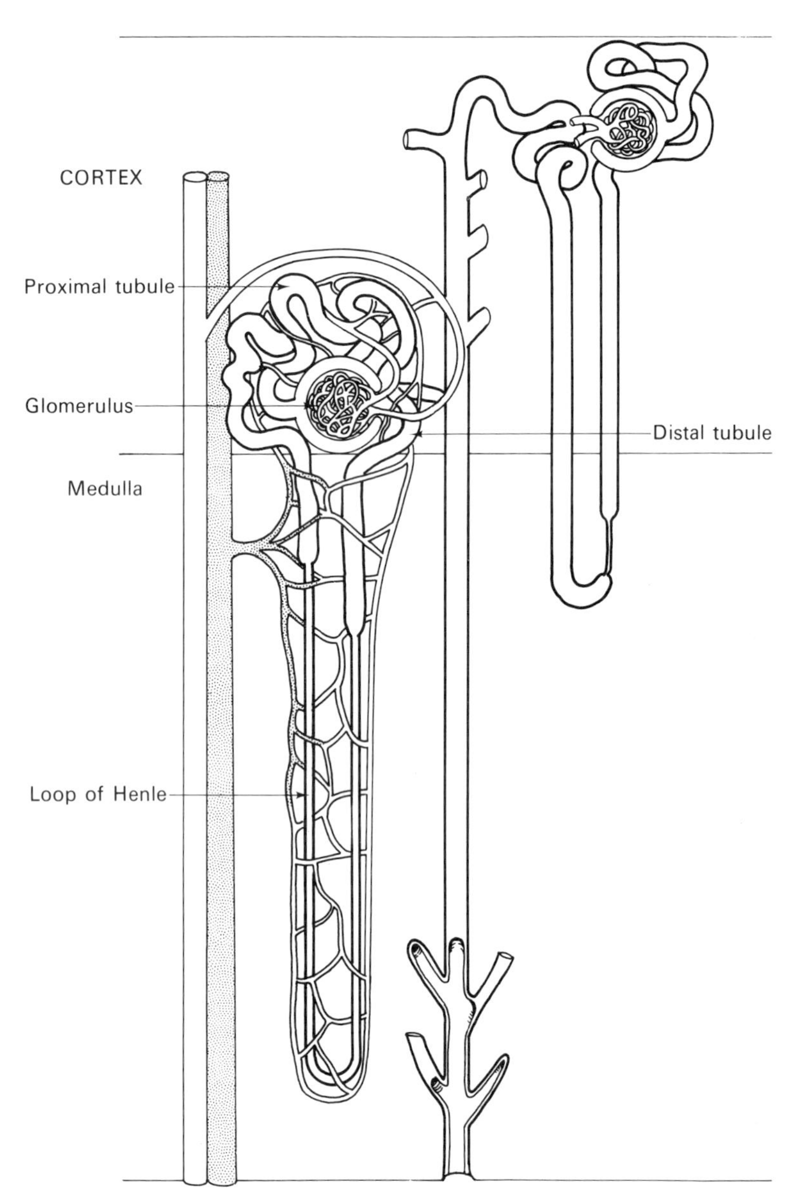

Fig. 4.3 Anatomy of a nephron.

Radiology of the urinary tract

Staight x-ray of the abdomen

This can be a very useful investigation in patients with renal failure. Often the outlines of each kidney are distinguishable, enabling their size, shape and position to be determined. Renal and ureteric calculi, the majority of which are radio-opaque, are usually readily visible.

Intravenous pyelogram (IVP)

This demonstrates the pelvis and calyces and is also helpful for showing the size, shape and position of the kidneys. In renal failure, high doses of the contrast medium have to be injected (high dose IVP). Using this method, in renal failure, it is possible to measure kidney size accurately and to detect any urinary tract obstruction, avoiding the need for retrograde pyelography.

Renal function

The most important function of the kidneys is to maintain the volume and composition of the body fluids within physiological limits by adjusting both the volume and the composition of the urine.

Functionally the kidney can be considered as a single nephron because the processes involved in urine formation, glomerular filtration, tubular reabsorption and tubular secretion are carried out in an identical manner in each one of them.

Glomerular filtration

Urine formation starts in the glomerulus by separation of a protein-free ultrafiltrate from the plasma. This filtered fluid (glomerular filtrate) then passes along the tubule where its composition and volume are greatly modified. Blood entering the glomerular capillaries has a pressure of 70 mmHg (9.3 kPa) (higher than in any other capillaries in the body), forcing fluid out into the glomerulus. This filtration pressure is opposed by the osmotic pressure of the plasma proteins 25 mmHg (3.3 kPa) and a back-pressure from within the nephron of 10 mmHg (1.3 kPa). The nett filtration pressure is therefore 35 mmHg (4.7 kPa).

A total of 170 litres of glomerular filtrate is produced each 24 hours, a value usually expressed in millilitres per minute as the glomerular filtration rate (GFR). The normal GFR is around 120 ml per minute and is very dependent on the state of the renal blood flow. A fall in renal blood flow reduces the filtration pressure in the glomerular capillaries and as a consequence the GFR is reduced.

Tubular absorption and secretion

The large volume of glomerular filtrate, having the same crystalloid composition as the plasma, is processed into urine by the action of the tubule. The total volume of filtrate when compared to a urine volume of only some 2–3 litres per day, with a very varied composition, demonstrates the magnitude of tubular activity. The main action of the tubules is to absorb water and solutes; normally over 99 per cent of the filtered water is absorbed before it reaches the ureters—85 per cent in the proximal and the remainder in the distal tubule. The latter is controlled by antidiuretic hormone (ADH). Failure to produce ADH, or failure of the cells to respond to it, causes diabetes insipidus.

The bulk of the filtered sodium is similarly absorbed in the proximal tubule along with the water. The remainder is absorbed in the distal tubule under the control of aldosterone.

Potassium is totally absorbed in the proximal tubule and its elimination is then by secretion in the distal tubule. The distal tubular cells also secrete hydrogen ions and can vary urinary pH anywhere in the range from 4.5 to 8.5.

Excretion of waste products

With the exception of carbon dioxide, all the waste products of metabolism are excreted in the urine. Those present in greatest amounts are urea, creatinine and various acid products of metabolism.

Urea

Urea is synthesized in the liver from ammonia that is released by amino acid breakdown. The quantity produced depends upon a number of factors: the protein intake, the body's need for amino acids, the rate of catabolism and the state of the liver. The normal level of urea in the plasma is 3.0–7.0 mmol/litre.

The plasma level is commonly used as an index of the GFR and is elevated in renal failure. An increase is not, however, specific to a deterioration in renal function and can also be caused by increased absorption or catabolism of proteins. Nevertheless, provided these possiblities are remembered, the plasma level of urea is a useful indicator of GFR.

Creatinine

Creatinine comes from muscle and the amount excreted is related to the muscle mass of the body and is not influenced by protein intake. The normal plasma level is 45–110 mmol/litre. Because it has a relatively constant rate of production and is eliminated exclusively by the kidney, changes in serum levels are directly related to GFR.

Creatinine clearance

The term 'clearance' is used as a measure of the smallest volume of plasma that would contain the total amount of a substance that is excreted in the urine. It therefore equals the amount of the substance excreted in urine per minute divided by the concentration of the substance in the plasma.

The clearance of a substance that is completely reabsorbed by the kidney, such as glucose, is zero. Substances that are not affected by the tubules have a clearance equal to the GFR.

In practice, the clearance of creatinine is a convenient method of measuring GFR. It has a constant plasma level, is not affected by the tubules and its excretion depends only on glomerular filtration.

Acid excretion

The kidneys have to secrete hydrogen ions because the metabolism of dietary protein produces about 70 mmol of non-volatile acid each day—mostly sulphuric and phosphoric acid. It is excreted in the urine as free acid (bound to phosphate compounds) and as ammonium. Failure of elimination leads to the metabolic acidosis of renal failure.

Water and electrolyte balance

The balance principle

The amount of any substance in a system at a particular time, provided it is not manufactured within the system, is determined by the difference between the quantity entering (the *input*) and that leaving (the *output*). When the input exceeds the output, the amount in the system increases—a state of positive balance. In the converse situation, with the output greater than the input, the amount in the system decreases—a state of negative balance. This very simple principle is fundamental to the understanding of fluid and electrolyte disorders.

Water balance

Input

An average adult ingests between 1500 and 3000 ml of water per day via the gastrointestinal tract—an amount that can be greatly increased in the face of excessive losses. Some water (about 300 ml) is produced in the body from the breakdown of foodstuffs.

Output

An average adult excretes between 600 and 2000 ml of water per day in the urine, controlled according to the amount of water in the body. The normal kidneys cannot reduce this excretion below 500 ml if all the waste products of metabolism are to be eliminated, for at this level the urine is maximally concentrated. This 'obligatory' urine volume is increased in patients whose rate of metabolism is increased.

Specific gravity is used to measure urinary concentration; normally it varies between 1.010 and 1.035. In patients in an ITU, however, specific gravity can be an inaccurate measure of concentration and tubular function, partly because of the difficulties of using a hydrometer in small volumes of urine and also because the presence of abnormal substances, protein, mannitol and dextrose affect concentration but have nothing to do with the kidneys' concentrating ability. Urine osmolality is a much better method in such patients and, where possible, should be compared to the plasma osmolality.

In addition to the urinary losses, at least 500 ml of water is lost via the lungs and a further 300 ml by evaporation (not sweating) from the skin. This total 'insensible loss' cannot be controlled and is increased considerably by hyperventilation and fever.

Losses through sweating can also be excessive with fever and in high environmental temperatures. The activity of the sweat glands is controlled via the sympathetic nervous system from the heat-regulating centre in the hypothalamus.

There is also a large daily turnover of fluid in the gastrointestinal tract, related to the secretion of the digestive juices. the bulk of this water is reabsorbed in the colon and only some 200 ml per day is lost in the faeces. Failure of reabsorption, for instance in diarrhoeal illnesses, may clearly lead to very large water losses.

Fluid balance charts that record only urinary losses are therefore poor guides to water balance and must always be interpreted by considering insensible losses in relation to each individual patient.

Regulation

Two mechanisms control the regulation of the volume and osmolality of the body fluids. They are the sensation of thirst, and the action of antidiuretic hormone (ADH) and aldosterone on the kidneys.

Thirst is caused by an increase in the osmolality of the ECF, which in turn stems from a negative water balance or the presence of an excessive quantity of solute. It is suppressed in the opposite circumstances.

An increase in ECF osmolality also stimulates the osmoreceptors in the hypothalamus and results in a release of ADH from the pituitary gland. The ADH acts on the distal kidney tubules and increases the reabsorption of water, diluting the blood and concentrating the urine. Once the osmolality of the ECF has returned to normal, the stimulus to ADH production is no longer present and the urinary output will adjust accordingly.

With a negative water balance the volume of the ECF is reduced and the associated hypovolaemia stimulates receptors in the kidneys that are concerned with blood volume control. These secrete renin which causes a release of aldosterone from the adrenal cortex. Aldosterone increases the reabsorption of sodium and water by the kidneys and the volume of ECF is returned towards normal.

Sodium balance

Input

Sodium enters the body by the gastrointestinal tract and is absorbed from the small intestine. The average daily intake is between 50 and 250 mmol. Forty per cent of the total body sodium is in the blood and interstitial fluid; the remainder is intracellular. The normal concentration in the blood is 132–145 mmol/litre.

Output

Sodium is secreted in sweat and in the gastrointestinal fluids. Most of that in the gastrointestinal tract is reabsorbed and normally only 10 mmol or less passes out in the faeces per day. As with water, massive amounts may be lost in gastrointestinal disease. It is excreted by the kidneys in amounts roughly equal to that ingested, less the amount lost in sweat; on average this urinary loss is between 100 and 240 mmol per 24 hours.

Regulation

Sodium is the major ion responsible for maintaining blood volume. The kidneys regulate its excretion according to body needs. Control is mediated by the renin–angiotensin–aldosterone system. Just as a low blood volume stimulates aldosterone release, a high blood volume suppresses it and there is a greater loss of sodium in the urine.

Potassium balance

Input

Potassium enters the body via the gastrointestinal tract and is absorbed from the small intestine; the average daily intake is between 50 and 150 mmol. Citrus fruits contain large amounts. Most of the body potassium is in the ICF but that present in the ECF has a marked influence on cardiac and neuromuscular function. The normal concentration in the blood is 3.3–4.5 mmol/litre. The high concentration gradient is maintained by active transport of potassium into cells and passive diffusion outwards.

Output

Small quantities of potassium are secreted in sweat and some into the gastrointestinal tract which again is a potential source of great losses in intestinal disease.

Ninety per cent of ingested potassium is excreted via the kidneys according to the state of the body's balance—on average between 35 and 90 mmol per 24 hours.

Regulation

The problem of potassium regulation is more complicated than that of sodium. Precise control rests with the kidneys and potassium elimination is closely related to the reabsorption of sodium and hydrogen ions.

Aldosterone increases the secretion of potassium in exchange for sodium. With an acidosis, potassium moves out of the cells in exchange for hydrogen ions and as a consequence more hydrogen ions are exchanged for sodium in the kidneys. In alkalosis, the reverse occurs and the serum potassium falls—hypokalaemic alkalosis. When glucose enters cells it takes potassium with it, an action that can be used to lower the serum potassium in acute hyperkalaemia.

5

Acid–Base

Acid–base physiology draws heavily and directly on certain disciplines of basic science, especially physical chemistry, so that it is essential to understand the form of terminology that is used.

Acid and base

The word 'acid' comes from the latin *acidus*, meaning sour-tasting. The term 'base' was introduced in 1774 by Rouelle who defined it as a substance that reacts with or neutralizes an acid to form a salt.

The misuse of these terms 'acid' and 'base' has since led to many difficulties and misunderstandings of acid–base balance in man and now the most widely accepted definition is that first proposed in 1923 by Brønsted and Lowry.

An *acid* is a substance capable of providing hydrogen ions (H^+) to the body.

A *base* is substance capable of accepting hydrogen ions (H^+).

A simple equation illustrating this is:

$$\underset{\text{(acid)}}{HB} \rightleftharpoons \underset{\text{(hydrogen ion)}}{H^+} + \underset{\text{(base)}}{B^-}$$

A strong acid is highly dissociated and provides many hydrogen ions; a weak acid is poorly dissociated, with few free hydrogen ions. The extent of the dissociation can be expressed quantitatively by a dissociation constant for that particular acid.

A strong base is likewise well dissociated and can accept many hydrogen ions; a weak base is poorly dissociated, accepting few hydrogen ions.

The pH scale

The concentration of H^+ in any solution can vary enormously and even in very acid solutions is very small, so the use of actual values is unwieldly and inconvenient. For this reason the pH scale, as first proposed by Sørensen in 1909, has been universally adopted to describe H^+ concentrations and the related degrees of 'acidity'.

The whole range of H^+ concentrations is described by simple numbers ranging between 0 and 14. This is made possible by the equation:

$$pH = \log_{10} \frac{1}{[H^+]} = -\log_{10} (H^+)$$

from which pH is defined as the negative common logarithm of the hydrogen ion concentration. It is negative so that the calculated pH values will be positive, as shown in the following example.

If a solution contains 4×10^{-8} mmol of hydrogen ions per litre

$$\begin{aligned} pH &= -\log (4 \times 10^{-8}) \\ &= -(\log 4 + \log 10^{-8}) \\ &= -(0.60 - 8.0) \\ &= -(-7.4) \\ &= 7.4 \end{aligned}$$

Note that because pH is the reciprocal of H^+ concentration, the stronger the acid the smaller is the pH value. Water is neutral with a pH of 7.

The disadvantage of the pH scale is that it is logarithmic and it is almost impossible to think in logarithms. It is helpful, however, to remember that a change of one pH unit represents a tenfold change in $[H^+]$, and a change of 0.3 pH unit a twofold change.

The pH of solutions containing both acids and bases is related to their respective concentrations and the dissociation constant (p*K*) of the acid. The relationship is expressed by the Henderson–Hasselbalch equation as:

$$pH = pK + \log \frac{(base)}{(acid)}$$

(p*K*: dissociation constant of the acid)

For blood this can be written as:

$$pH = pK + \log \frac{\textit{bicarbonate}\ (HCO_3^-)}{\textit{carbonic acid}\ (H_2CO_3)}$$

(p*K*: dissociation constant of carbonic acid)

The p*K* of carbonic acid is 6.1 and the ratio of bicarbonate to carbonic acid in blood is 20:1. The pH of blood is therefore

$$\begin{aligned} &= 6.1 + \log_{20} \\ &= 6.1 + 1.3 \\ &= 7.4 \end{aligned}$$

The normal range of blood pH is 7.36–7.44.

The Henderson–Hasselbalch equation can also be stated in a slightly different form as:

$$pH = 6.1 + \log \frac{(HCO_3^-)}{(P_{CO_2} \times 0.03)}$$

(0.03 is the solubility co-efficient of carbon dioxide)

which serves to highlight the relationship that exists between carbon dioxide and carbonic acid.

Regulation of blood pH

Normally the pH of blood is maintained within the narrow limits of 7.36–7.44 by a number of inter-related processes involving the blood buffers, the lungs and the kidneys. Were it not for these the blood would quickly become acid; ingested food produces H^+ during its metabolism and carbon dioxide is continually entering the blood as an end-product of carbohydrate and fat metabolism.

Blood buffers

These provide a remarkably efficient short-term defence and enable hydrogen ions to be transported from their site of production to their site of elimination with a minimum alteration in the blood pH.

The principal blood buffer systems are:

(1) the bicarbonate system

$$HCO_3^- + H^+ \rightleftharpoons H_2CO_3 \rightleftharpoons H_2O + CO_2$$

(2) the phosphate system

$$HPO_4^- + H^+ \rightleftharpoons H_2PO_4^-$$

(3) the protein system (especially haemoglobin)

$$Protein^- + H^+ \rightleftharpoons HPr$$

The bicarbonate buffer system, which is the most important in the extracellular fluid, buffers hydrogen ions to form carbonic acid (H_2CO_3), a volatile acid which dissociates to H_2O and CO_2 and is then eliminated by the lungs.

Whilst the buffer systems provide effective temporary protection, hydrogen ions from acids other than carbonic can be eliminated only by renal excretion.

The contribution of the plasma proteins to the buffer capacity of the blood is small, but that of haemoglobin is very important because it is present in the erythrocytes which are the main site of carbonic acid formation. It is therefore readily available to buffer hydrogen ions derived from carbonic acid. Proteins are also probably the most important buffers in other cells.

Excretion of acid

Lungs
The respiratory centre is sensitive to changes in pH and is stimulated by a fall in pH. This causes hyperventilation and an increased rate of excretion of carbon dioxide (carbonic acid).

Kidneys
The kidneys regulate blood pH by the proximal and distal tubular secretion of hydrogen ions formed in the tubular cell by the action of carbonic anhydrase. This process leads to the renal excretion of hydrogen ions and the regeneration of bicarbonate ions which diffuse back into the blood to replenish the buffer system.

Very few of the hydrogen ions appear in the urine 'free' because they are buffered by bases present in the glomerular filtrate or secreted by the tubules.

Elimination by the kidneys is a relatively slow process (24–36 hours) compared to the rapid elimination (a few minutes) by the lungs.

Alkalosis and acidosis

An increase in blood pH above 7.4 constitutes an *alkalosis*, and a decrease below this value an *acidosis*. Since the p*K* value is a constant, the ways in which either of these two conditions might arise can be appreciated by studying the 'tail' of the Henderson–Hasselbalch equation, that is the ratio of bicarbonate to carbon dioxide.

For example, an increase in carbon dioxide tension as occurs in ventilatory failure, reduces the value of the ratio and hence the pH decreases giving an acidosis of respiratory origin—*respiratory acidosis*. Conversely, a decrease in carbon dioxide tension by hyperventilation increases the value of the ratio and elevates the pH, giving an alkalosis of respiratory origin—*respiratory alkalosis*.

The bicarbonate concentration is changed primarily by metabolic processes that affect the acid content of the body. A decrease in bicarbonate occurs when there is excess acid, as in shock where lactic acid production is increased. This decreases the value of the ratio and the pH falls, causing an acidosis of metabolic origin—*metabolic acidosis*.

An increase in bicarbonate concentration, perhaps due to the administration of sodium bicarbonate or secondary to the loss of acid from the stomach, increases the pH, producing an alkalosis of metabolic origin—*metabolic alkalosis*.

Some of the common causes of acid–base disturbances are shown in Table 5.1.

Table 5.1 Common causes of acid-base disturbances

Metabolic	Respiratory
Acidosis	
1. Over production of acids: Shock, cardiac arrest, diabetic ketosis.	*Ventilatory failure of any cause*
2. Impaired renal excretion of acid: acute and chronic renal failure.	
3. Ingestion of acids for example NH_4Cl.	
4. Loss of bicarbonate-rich intestinal secretions.	
Alkalosis	
1. Loss of gastric acid; Vomiting Naso-gastric suction.	Any cause of hyperventilation.
2. Provision of excess base Blood transfusion (citrate metabolized to base) Sodium Bicarbonate.	

Two further points require mention. First, an acidosis or alkalosis may have a *mixed* cause, as for example when shock and ventilatory failure coexist and produce both a respiratory and a metabolic acidosis. Secondly, an acidosis or alkalosis may be *compensated* when secondary changes in pulmonary or renal function have restored the pH to normal by returning the value of the ratio to normal. In renal failure, for example, there is a decrease in the bicarbonate concentration resulting from the retention of acid products of metabolism. This initially causes a metabolic acidosis, but because the fall in pH stimulates the respiratory centre, causing hyperventilation, the carbon dioxide tension also falls and the pH returns to normal; the acidosis is said to be compensated.

Relationship between hydrogen ions and potassium ions

Hydrogen ions and potassium ions are closely inter-related in the intra- and extracellular fluid. Disturbances in the balance of one of them can produce changes in the other.

1. Acidosis leads to potassium depletion; the accumulation of hyd-

rogen ions in tissue cells displaces potassium ions into the extracellular fluid from which they are lost in the urine. Initially there is an increase in the serum potassium.

2. Alkalosis leads to potassium depletion because hydrogen ions are not available for exchange with sodium ions in the kidney; potassium ions are exchanged instead and potassium is lost in the urine.

3. Potassium depletion leads to an alkalosis in the extracellular fluid because the intracellular potassium is partly replaced by hydrogen ions. There is therefore an intracellular acidosis associated with the extracellular alkalosis.

Measurement of the acid–base status

Using samples of arterial blood pH, $P\text{CO}_2$, bicarbonate concentration and base excess are determined.

Plasma bicarbonate

The normal value of plasma bicarbonate is 21–26 mmol/litre but it is influenced by the carbon dioxide content of the blood. To eliminate this respiratory variation the level can be measured with the carbon dioxide tension of the sample fixed at the normal value of 40 mmHg (5.3 kPa). This figure is the *standard bicarbonate*.

Base excess

This is defined as the number of moles of acid or base that are required to restore one litre of blood to a pH of 7.4 while the $P\text{CO}_2$ is held constant at 40 mmHg (5.3 kPa). The value is therefore helpful in quantifying the metabolic component of an acid–base disturbance. Under normal conditions it is zero. With a metabolic acidosis, alkali (bicarbonate) will have to be added to the blood to restore the pH and the result is expressed as a negative value, better referred to as a base deficit. In a metabolic alkalosis it has a positive value and is rightly described as a base excess.

The base deficit is a convenient figure for calculating the dose of sodium bicarbonate required to correct a metabolic acidosis. For example, if the extracellular fluid volume constitutes one-fifth of the body weight then, with a base deficit of –6, the number of millimoles of sodium bicarbonate required to correct the acidosis is equal to:

$$\text{Base deficit} \times 0.2 \times \text{body weight in kg}$$

$$6 \times 0.2 \times 75\ \text{kg} = 90\ \text{mmol}$$

Interpretation of acid–base results

The normal values are:

pH	7.40 (± 0.05)
P_{CO_2}	40 (± 5) mmHg (5.3 ± 0.6 kPa)
Standard bicarbonate	22–26 mmol/litre
Base excess (BE)	(± 3) mmol/litre

An approach to the abnormal result

The analysis of the results must be made in a sequential manner as follows.

1. Is there an acidosis of alkalosis (remember the possibility of compensation)?

A pH less than 7.4 = acidosis
A pH greater than 7.4 = alkalosis

If the pH is 7.4, are the values of the standard bicarbonate and the P_{CO_2} normal? If they are abnormal, then some compensation has taken place.

2. Is the disturbance metabolic or respiratory?

For an acidosis, if the P_{CO_2} is elevated, it is respiratory; if the standard bicarbonate is reduced or there is a base deficit, it is metabolic.

For an alkalosis the changes are in the opposite direction.

The following are some examples.

pH	7.22	7.23
P_{CO_2}	75	14
Standard bicarbonate	24	17
Base excess	0	−20

1. Acidosis present
2. Disturbance is respiratory because the P_{CO_2} is elevated; standard bicarbonate and base excess are normal.

1. Acidosis present.
2. Disturbance is metabolic because the standard bicarbonate is low and the base excess negative.
3. The low P_{CO_2} is due to stimulation of the respiratory centre by the acidosis and is an attempt at respiratory compensation of the metabolic acidosis.

pH	7.52	7.50
$P\text{CO}_2$	27	43
Standard bicarbonate	25	43
Base excess	+1	+9

1. Alkalosis.
2. Disturbance is respiratory because the $P\text{CO}_2$ is low. Standard bicarbonate and base excess are within normal limits

1. Alkalosis.
2. Disturbance is metabolic because the standard bicarbonate and base excess are high and the $P\text{CO}_2$ is within normal limits.

pH	7.39
$P\text{CO}_2$	26
Standard bicarbonate	18
Base excess	−8

1. pH normal but does it represent a compensated state?
2. Yes, because $P\text{CO}_2$ and standard bicarbonate are abnormal.
3. Is it a compensated respiratory alkalosis or a compensated metabolic acidosis? Cannot say without clinical details.

Pitfalls in analysis

As with all other investigations, the results should be looked at in relation to the patient's condition. If they appear anomalous then consider:

1. was the sample arterial?
2. was there delay in analysing the sample?
3. did the patient hyperventilate when the sample was being taken?
4. is the patient's temperature normal?

All of these will clearly affect the results.

Technique of arterial puncture

The common sites for taking a sample of arterial blood are the radial artery at the wrist, the brachial artery in the antecubital fossa and the femoral artery in the groin. In each situation the course of the artery must be defined by placing the left middle and index fingers along the line of maximal pulsation. The needle is introduced between the two fingers and advanced slowly. Arterial blood should enter the heparinized syringe easily and should pulsate. After taking the sample, all air bubbles must be removed and then the end of the syringe can be sealed. The syringe should be gently rolled between the hands to ensure that the sample is properly mixed with the heparin. If there is any delay before analysis, the sample must be kept in ice.

Firm pressure must be applied over the puncture site for at least five minutes; otherwise, large and unsightly haematomas may form.

Treatment of acid–base disturbances

Changes in pH produce their effects by altering the rate of enzyme action in various physiological systems. In the great majority of cases the essential treatment is to correct the underlying circulatory, metabolic or respiratory disturbance. However, in certain acute situations, it may be necessary to correct a severe metabolic acidosis (pH less than 7.1) with intravenous sodium bicarbonate. This should be given in a dose obtained from the formula given previously.

Metabolic alkalosis rarely requires treatment. In an ITU patient it is often an indication of hypokalaemia and the pH will return towards normal with potassium replacement. Ammonium chloride should not be used.

6
Metabolism

Metabolism

Metabolism consists of two opposite processes, anabolism and catabolism, proceeding simultaneously.

Anabolism is the synthesis of body constituents as during growth and tissue repair.

Catabolism is the breakdown of body constituents for the provision of energy.

At any one time the overall metabolic balance depends upon their respective rates; if anabolism is greater than catabolism there is a positive metabolic balance, and if catabolism exceeds anabolism the balance is negative.

Normal energy requirements

In health, energy is required for a variety of purposes: the performance of external work, the muscular movements of the heart and respiration, the maintenance of body temperature and the various synthetic processes associated with cell growth and replacement. Not surprisingly, with so many variable demands, the 'normal' requirement is difficult to define and varies over a wide range—reflecting, amongst other things, the degree of physical activity, body size and changes in environmental temperature.

Basal or resting energy requirements are often expressed in relation to the surface area of the body, and the basal metabolic rate (BMR) is the energy required per square metre per hour; it is of the order of 40 calories, that is 1728 calories per day for a person with a surface area of 1.8 m^2. Requirements for work and exercise are extra to this basal figure; for a sedentary person the daily needs are around 2700 calories and for a heavy manual worker approximately 3800 calories.

Energy requirements during illness

In critical illness and following injury there is a major increase in the rate of catabolism, more so if infection and fever are present. This increase is partly brought about by changes in the normal hormonal control of metabolism; the levels of adrenaline, hydrocortisone, growth hormone and glucagon are all elevated and each one stimulates catabolism. In addition, they oppose the action of the anabolic hormone insulin and therefore retard anabolism.

The energy demands are proportional to the severity of the disturbance; a severely burnt patient uses between 5000 and 6000 calories and one with pneumonia around 4000 calories. If insufficient calories are supplied to meet these demands, the body uses its own limited calorie sources and then has to break down protein to provide energy. A high rate of catabolism is therefore associated with a rapid disintegration of body protein and a negative protein balance; such patients lose weight and are susceptible to a number of serious complications.

Provision of energy

All the body's energy is ultimately derived from the breakdown (oxidation) of foodstuffs to carbon dioxide and water. The oxidation of fat provides 9 calories per gram, carbohydrate 4 calories per gram, protein 4 calories per gram and alcohol 7 calories per gram. The energy value of any food can therefore be calculated if its constituents are known.

Metabolism of foodstuffs

The pathways and processes by which carbohydrates, fats and proteins are metabolized are closely inter-related and many of the reactions are influenced by circulating hormones.

Carbohydrate metabolism (Fig. 6.1)

Carbohydrates are absorbed predominantly as glucose; small amounts of fructose and galactose are absorbed but are converted to glucose in the liver. Limited quantities of carbohydrate are stored as glycogen in the liver and muscles. Muscle glycogen provides the energy necessary for muscular contraction but is not available to replenish the blood glucose. Liver glycogen is converted to blood glucose and the store can maintain a normal blood level for up to 24 hours of starvation, after which fats and proteins are used as energy sources. If the glycogen stores are full, any surplus glucose is converted to fat and stored in the fat depots. The tissues obtain glucose from the blood, and the central nervous system in particular is highly dependent on blood glucose; sustained hypoglycaemia may result in cerebral damage.

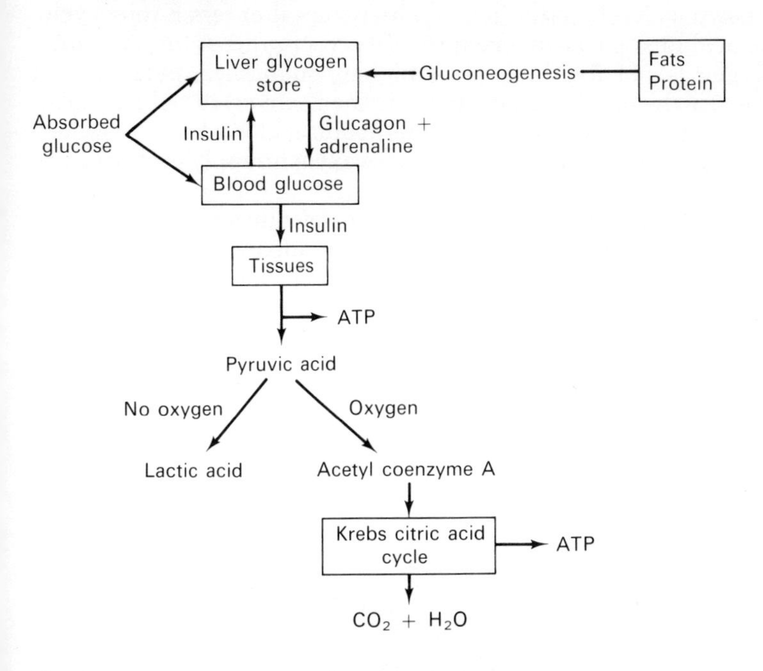

Fig. 6.1 Pathways of carbohydrate metabolism.

Regulation of the blood glucose

The balance between the storage and utilization of glucose is adjusted according to need and is controlled by a number of hormones, notably insulin.

When the blood glucose rises above normal levels, as after a meal, increased amounts of insulin are secreted from the beta cells of the islets of Langerhans and promote the formation of glycogen and the utilization of glucose. Conversely, when the blood glucose level falls and the insulin secretion is reduced, liver glycogen is converted to glucose; this process, glycogenolysis, is facilitated by glucagon secreted from the alpha cells of the islets of Langerhans and adrenaline secreted from the adrenal medulla. Should the liver store be depleted, additional glucose can be synthesized from protein and fat, a process known as gluconeogenesis.

Conversion of glucose to energy (glycolysis)
The tissues derive energy from glucose by breaking it down in two stages. The first stage is anaerobic (that is, it does not require oxygen) and through this glucose is converted to pyruvic acid. The second stage is aerobic (that is, it requires oxygen) and the pyruvic acid is degraded to carbon dioxide and water via a series of chemical reactions known as Krebs' citric acid cycle. Before it enters Krebs' cycle, pyruvic acid has to be converted to acetyl coenzyme A (acetyl CoA).

If oxygen is not available in sufficient quantities, pyruvic acid cannot enter the aerobic stage and it is then converted to lactic acid. This reaction is the reason for the metabolic acidosis that is encountered in conditions (such as shock) where oxygen supply to the tissues is reduced.

The energy produced in the two stages of glucose breakdown is stored as 'high-energy' phosphate bonds in adenosine triphosphate (ATP). With the release of energy, ATP loses one of the phosphate bonds to form adenosine diphosphate (ADP).

Fat metabolism (Fig. 6.2)

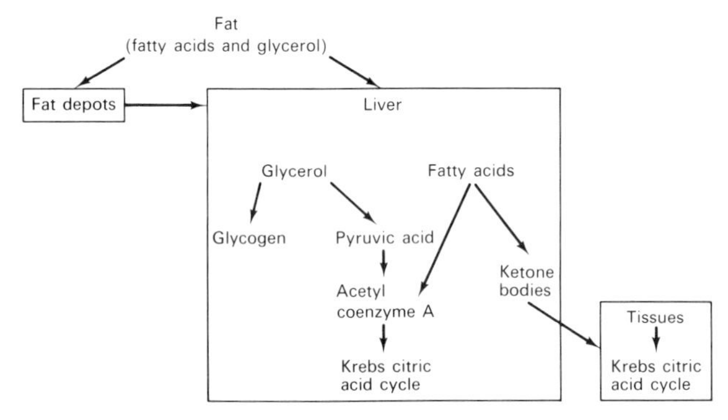

Fig. 6.2 Pathways of fat metabolism.

Fats are absorbed as fatty acids and glycerol which, when they are not immediately required for the provision on energy, are stored in the fat depots (subcutaneous and retroperitoneal tissues) as neutral fat. The energy reserves in the fat depots far exceed those of the liver glycogen.

The fats are mobilized, as required, from the depots and transported to the liver where they are initially broken down to glycerol and fatty acids. The glycerol enters the first stage of glycolysis and may be converted to either glycogen or pyruvic acid. The fatty acids are converted to acetyl CoA which then enters Krebs' cycle (cf. carbohydrate metabolism) to provide energy.

The essential components of Krebs' cycle are, however, derived from carbohydrate metabolism and if they are inadequate, as in starvation, or abnormal, as in diabetes mellitus, the cycle does not function and acetyl CoA cannot be metabolized normally. When this happens the molecules of acetyl CoA combine together in pairs, in the liver, to form the keto acids, acetoacetic acid and beta-hydroxybutyric acid, which can be utilized by other tissues to provide energy. An excess of keto acids in the blood causes a metabolic acidosis.

Protein metabolism (Fig. 6.3)

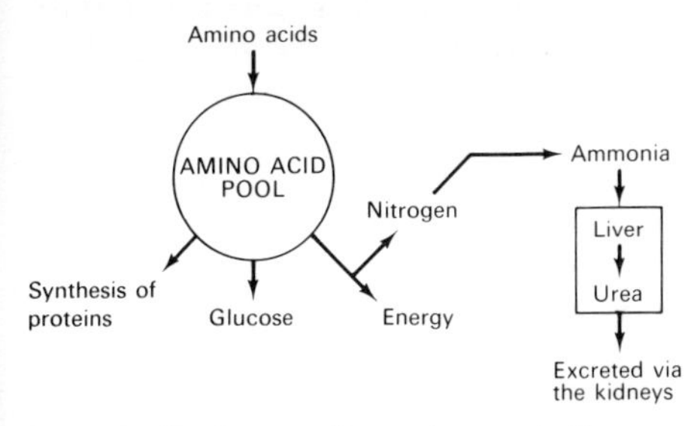

Fig. 6.3 Pathways of protein metabolism.

Proteins are absorbed as amino acids, and enter a common amino acid 'pool' in the blood and tissues. From this they are used for the formation of tissue proteins, plasma proteins, hormones and nucleic acids. The amino acid pool is in a continual state of flux with amino acids being added, transformed or removed. Many amino acids can be synthesized in the body by transformation from other amino acids or from pyruvic acid, but there is a group of eight amino acids which cannot be synthesized and they are termed 'essential', meaning that they are essential foodstuffs. Surplus amino acids are converted into carbon dioxide and water, with the release of energy and the formation of urea.

The nitrogen from the amino acids forms ammonia which is then converted in the liver to urea by a series of chemical reactions known as Krebs' urea cycle. Production of urea is therefore increased as the rate of protein breakdown increases. In severe liver disease the liver is unable to form the urea from ammonia and the blood levels are low.

As already mentioned, in these states of high calorie demand body proteins are broken down for energy purposes. Urea production and nitrogen loss is high, and unless sufficient calories and nitrogen are provided a negative nitrogen balance develops.

Metabolic role of the liver

The liver clearly has an essential role in the metabolism of the three major foodstuffs.

1. It stores glucose as glycogen, the breakdown of which contributes to the maintenance of the blood glucose.
2. It forms keto acids when fat is being metabolized in the absence of sufficient carbohydrates.
3. It forms urea from ammonia.

In addition, the liver is the source of plasma albumin, fibrinogen and most of the coagulation factors. It also has an important role in metabolizing drugs and detoxifying many noxious substances. Not surprisingly, abnormalities of liver function can produce widespread metabolic derangements.

7

Monitoring

The physiological status of critically ill patients changes in many rapid and subtle ways which often cannot be detected by the traditional forms of bedside observation. The changes occur too quickly and they are often only apparent in 'signals' that cannot be sensed by hand. The development of instrumentation for patient monitoring has overcome many of these limitations and its use is now an integral and essential part of intensive therapy.

Patient monitoring equipment

This detects and displays physiological information and may warn of impending crises. The total pattern of information is formed by collation of a number of individual physiological variables or 'signals' that can be monitored automatically. In a particular patient it is always necessary to select for monitoring those signals (Table 7.1) that have direct clinical relevance in contradistinction to the many that can be technically acquired.

Table 7.1 'Signals'

Cardiovascular system:	Electrocardiogram (ECG)
	Arterial pressure
	Central venous pressure (CVP)
	Pulmonary capillary wedge pressure
	Direct left atrial pressure
	Cardiac output
Respiratory system:	Rate and rhythm of respiration
	Arterial blood gases
Renal and electrolyte system:	Urinary output
	Serum electrolytes
Central nervous system:	Electroencephalogram (EEG)
	Intracranial pressure
Body temperature:	Rectal temperature
	Skin temperature

Elements of a monitoring system

Irrespective of the actual signal, all monitoring systems are formed from the same basic elements (Fig. 7.1).

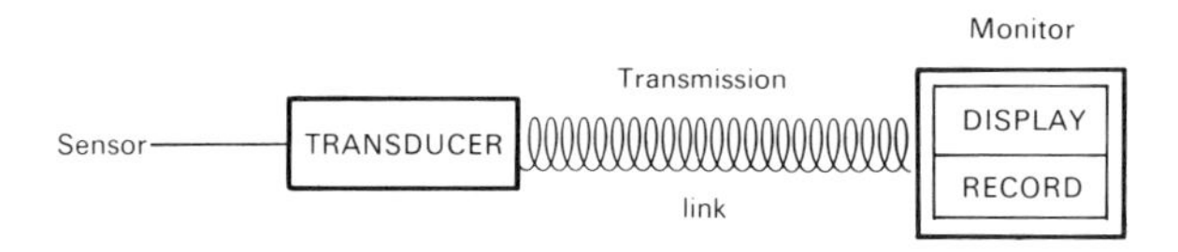

Fig. 7.1 The basic elements of a monitoring system.

1. A sensor to detect the signal.
2. A transducer to convert the signal, where necessary, into an electrical form.
3. A transmission link to carry the signal, from the sensor or transducer, to the monitor.
4. A monitor to process, display and record the signal.

Individual signals

Electrocardiogram

The ECG is universally monitored in every ITU. It originates from the heart in an electrical form and therefore a transducer is unnecessary.

It is sensed by skin electrodes placed on the chest or, where this is not possible. on the shoulders or limbs. The majority of ECG electrodes are now disposable and vary in appearance according to the manufacturer. Each consists of a central metal disc (the electrode), usually made of silver and silver chloride, surrounded by an adhesive ring of tape or porous foam rubber (Fig. 7.2). When fixing them to the skin, electrical contact is improved by using a conducting paste or jelly. The ECG cable is attached to the electrode by a press-stud, a wire connector or a crocodile clip.

When choosing a particular design of electrode for use in an ITU it is necessary to consider:

1. the ease and speed of application;
2. the quality of ECG signal obtained;
3. the suitability for long-term monitoring;
4. the type of connector;
5. the cost.

Ease and speed of application are essential because the electrodes may have to be attached during situations of emergency where an

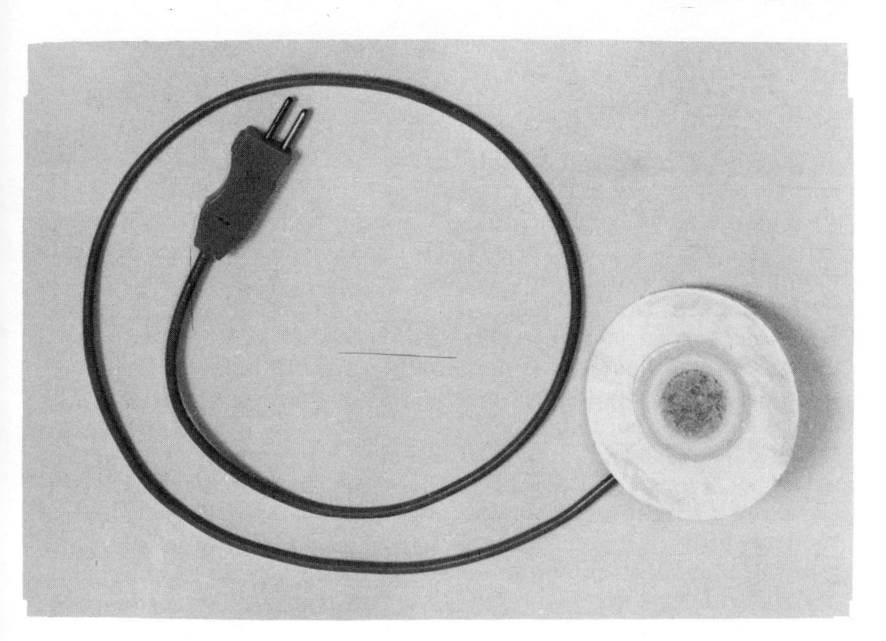

Fig. 7.2 An ECG electrode.

immediate display of the ECG is imperative. Some electrodes are provided with conductive jelly already present (pre-jelled) and this avoids the often somewhat messy application of jelly from a tube. Once in place they have to maintain close contact with the skin, sometimes for several days. The metal must therefore be inert and non-irritant and the overall design rugged with strong connectors that can withstand long-term monitoring without breaking.

The longer the electrodes are in place, the more likely are skin reactions to develop. These range from mild erythema to frank ulceration and are usually caused by the adhesive backing material. Light-weight micropore tape or porous foam are the most suitable materials for minimizing this complication; they are non-irritating and have a low allergy potential.

The total size of the electrodes has to be limited so that when in place they do not interfere with examination of the chest or the use of defibrillator paddles, nor should they obscure too large an area on a chest x-ray.

Cost is a most important consideration and varies between different manufacturers. Since electrodes are the 'vital link' in the monitoring system, the price and performance need to be balanced accordingly.

Intravascular pressures

These are sensed by indwelling arterial or venous catheters which are connected to transducers to convert the pressure into an electrical voltage. Cannulation of a radial artery is preferred for arterial pressure monitoring; the brachial artery may be used but the femoral artery is unsuitable because of the risks of infection. For accurate monitoring, the catheter must remain patent; thrombus formation in its lumen or kinking will cause a loss or dampening of the signal.

Normal pressure waveforms should be sharply defined with rapid upstrokes and clear peaks and troughs. When 'damped' these features are less obvious, and the height of the pressure falls (Fig. 7.3). The tendency to thrombus formation is greatest with arterial catheters because the relatively high pressure forces blood back into the catheter. The likelihood of this happening can be reduced by inserting a continuous infusion device (Intraflow) between the catheter and the transducer. This is connected to a 500 ml bag of fluid that has a Fenwall blood infusion pump inflated around it to a pressure of 300 mmHg which overcomes the pressure in the arterial system (Fig. 7.4). It allows a small (3–5 ml/hour), but constant, flow of heparinized saline to pass along the catheter. At this flow rate the quantity of fluid and heparin administered is minimal.

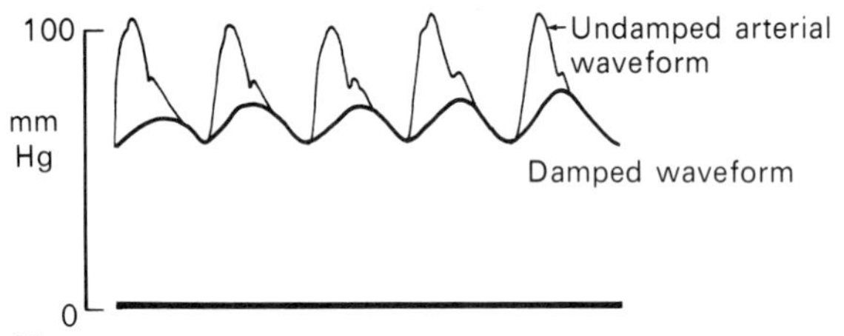

Fig. 7.3 Normal and damped arterial pressure waveforms.

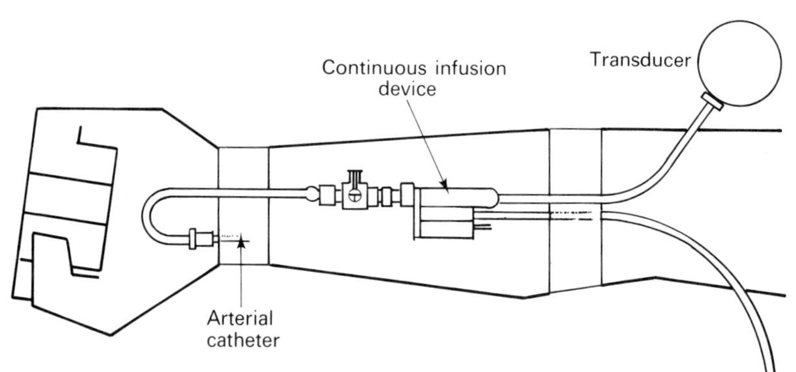

Fig. 7.4 A continuous infusion and flushing system.

Pressure transducers vary in design and size (Fig. 7.5); some are small and can be attached to the patient, whilst larger varieties have to be mounted on a separate table. They all operate on the same principle. A diaphragm inside the transducer is stretched by the pressure; this alters its electrical characteristics and so changes the voltage output from the transducer.

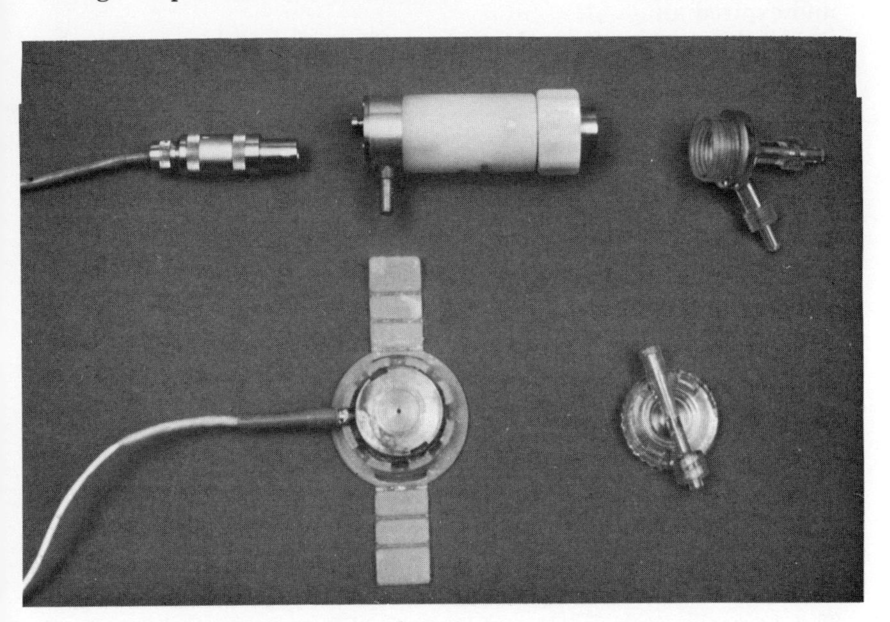

Fig. 7.5 A variety of pressure transducers.

Before use, each transducer must be calibrated against a known pressure source, usually a column of mercury. It is then possible to equate the voltage output from the transducer with mmHg; the calibration needs to be repeated at frequent intervals. When reading vascular pressures the transducer must always be at the same level (zero reference level) with respect to the patient. It is useless to compare measurements that are made with the patient in different positions.

Arterial pressure can also be measured automatically by using sphygmomanometers with self-inflating cuffs. The times of inflation can be varied and the levels of systolic and diastolic pressure are sensed by either a microphone, which detects the Korotkoff sounds, or an ultrasonic device, which detects arterial wall movement or blood flow. These units are very useful, particularly in paediatric intensive therapy.

Respiratory rate and rhythm

These can be sensed in a number of different ways by the following.

1. A temperature sensitive device (thermistor), placed in the nostril, which detects the difference in temperature between inspired and expired air.

2. A strain gauge around the chest. Stretching of the gauge during inspiration affects its electrical resistance and each breath can be detected.

3. An impedance method which measures the electrical resistance, across the chest, to a high frequency electrical current. This changes from inspiration to expiration and respiration can be recorded.

None of these methods measures the size of each breath and they are used mainly for monitoring the respiratory pattern of deeply comatose patients at risk from sudden respiratory arrest.

Apnoea monitors are used in neonatal intensive therapy for monitoring premature babies with respiratory, neurological and metabolic problems. The apnoea mattress is a sectional mattress that fits under the sheet in a cot or incubator. As the baby breathes, this movement results in puffs of air coming from the different segments. The puffs are detected by a thermistor and converted into audible clicks. These cease if the movements of respiration stop.

Continuous monitoring of arterial P_{O_2}

This is used mainly in neonatal practice but has some application in adult intensive therapy. Two techniques have been developed.

1. An intra-arterial catheter containing an oxygen sensitive electrode is placed in the umbilical artery.

2. A cutaneous oxygen electrode is placed on the skin. With good skin circulation the readings from this correlate with the arterial P_{O_2}.

Electroencephalogram (EEG)

The EEG is a low amplitude electrical signal sensed from the brain by numerous electrodes placed on the scalp. These have to be positioned very carefully by sticking them to cleansed areas of the scalp with colloidin. Electrode jelly is then forced through a hole in the electrode by means of a blunt needle attached to a syringe.

For continuous monitoring of cerebral function a modified EEG can be sensed from two scalp electrodes. This method is of value in the management of patients with hepatic coma and during open-heart surgery.

Body temperature

This can be monitored continuously from the skin and rectum by electrical methods. It has general application but is especially useful in managing patients suffering from induced or accidental hypothermia and following cardiac surgery.

The monitor

This processes the various signals and displays them on a screen. The monitor may be single- or multi-channel, that is it can accept one or several signals. In ITUs the multi-channel types are essential and are adapted to monitor ECG, vascular pressures, body temperature and, sometimes, respiration. Each signal is processed in a separate compartment of the monitor (module) and these can be changed and removed without affecting the other modules—a great advantage when maintenance and repair become necessary.

Electronically, a module contains an amplifier which increases the size of the signal and can sometimes be varied by an external control (gain control). ECG modules also contain a filter which removes certain electrical frequencies, particularly the 50 Hz of the electrical mains, that can interfere with the signal.

The display is some form of oscilloscope screen. Originally oscilloscope screens were coated with a certain coloured phosphor which glowed as the waveform passed across the screen. This had two disadvantages, the trace faded and only short lengths were visible at any one time and also the phosphor 'burnt' leaving permanent marks across the screen. This method has now been superseded by the use of 'memory' scopes which store the electrical waveform behind the screen and flash it on and off the screen at a rate sufficient to create the appearance of a continuous wave. The problems of fading and burning are eliminated, and also the trace can be 'frozen' on the screen for detailed study or to retain some change of particular interest.

If permanent records are required, the monitor has to be linked to a chart or tape recorder.

Alarm systems

These can be incorporated into the monitor to provide an alarm should the value of a particular variable deviate outside certain limits. They are most often used for heart rate. When the limits are breached, an alarm (in the form of a flashing light or audible sounds) is emitted to attract the attention of a member of staff. When properly used, these systems make a worthwhile practical contribution but often they are abused and many avoidable false alarms occur.

Artefacts in patient monitoring

Artefacts represent some form of unwanted interference in the acquired signals. They can originate from the patient or any part of the monitoring system and may be severe enough to completely mask a signal. With electrodes any form of patient movement, shivering or muscle tremor can cause them; if the electrodes are not applied properly they may pick up the 50 Hz frequency from the mains supplying the power from the many kinds of equipment in use around the patient.

Catheters may become blocked or kinked or flick around inside a vessel such as the pulmonary artery. Artefacts may be due to electrical faults in the monitor itself but technology has become very reliable and the great majority arise, as indicated, from the 'patient/sensor interface', emphasizing the need for meticulous care to this link in the monitoring chain.

Computers and patient monitoring

In a small number of ITUs computers are used to analyse, store and record the large amounts of physiological information provided by monitoring systems. They have not proved to be universally successful and their 'routine' place in intensive therapy has yet to be established.

Electrical safety

The use in ITUs of many kinds of electrical equipment, linked in some way to the patients, creates a potential danger of electrocution should some electrical fault develop. Current leakages to patients with intracardiac and intravascular catheters need only be very small (microamps) to produce ventricular fibrillation. Nursing staff must be acutely aware of this hazard and immediately report to the technician responsible any apparent faults in the equipment. They should observe certain simple safety procedures (Table 7.2).

Table 7.2 Simple safety procedures

1.	Inspect equipment for damage before plugging it in
2.	Report any defects to the technician
3.	Keep fluids away from equipment and cables
4.	Take care when plugging and unplugging equipment
5.	Never ignore a tingling sensation when touching a piece of equipment

Every ITU must have a planned rota for routinely inspecting and checking all monitoring equipment and electrical outlets. Faulty earth connections are especially dangerous.

Manufacturers have to comply to very stringent safety codes. The safety standards are now very high but have increased the cost of the equipment.

Laboratory equipment

ITUs, whilst having close contacts with the main hospital laboratories, should have their own laboratory. It is unreasonable and impractical to expect the 24 hour a day, 7 day a week demand (much of which falls outside normal working hours) to be fully catered for by a centralized hospital service. The unit laboratory must have its own flame photometer to measure electrolytes, a blood gas analyser and a reflectance meter to measure blood sugar. Additions to this limited yet basic range can be made in accordance with the demands of the unit.

Section B
Nursing practice

8

Unit administration and organization

Successful nursing management of an ITU is founded on the nurse's meticulous attention to detail and her conscientious routine care of the patient. For this to be achieved the unit must have an adequate and appropriately structured nursing establishment with additional provisions for teaching and training.

Continuity of care stems from the routine organization of patient care linked with the recording and charting of observations. The functions and activities of an ITU produce stresses for the patients, their relatives and its staff; ways of reducing these depend on effective staff communication.

Nursing establishment

To provide constant care and attention for each patient, the number of trained nurses required has to be based on the ratio of one nurse for each patient for each of the three shifts throughout the 24 hours. When the necessary allowances for training, holiday and sick leave have been made, this means 4.25 nurses per bed; that is, for an eight-bedded unit, an establishment of 34 nurses. This figure needs to be reviewed each time nurses are given an increase in their holiday entitlement or a reduction in the number of working hours.

The staffing consists of nurses of varying seniority (Fig. 8.1) from nursing officer to student nurse. Ideally the pre-registered students are not counted as part of the total complement. Of the qualified nurses, approximately 20 per cent should be experienced sisters and at least 40 per cent experienced staff nurses. Of the remainder one-half may be gaining clinical experience and one-half undertaking a post-registration course. It is important to keep a larger balance of experienced staff in order to provide adequate supervision for the inexperienced nurse who needs to learn and accept responsibility gradually.

To maintain a constant standard of nursing care there has to be a sufficient number of nurses throughout the 24 hours. They must be allocated in equal numbers to each shift because there is little, or no, variation between the day and night workload. At times, when the unit is quiet, the number of nurses on duty may be excessive. These periods should, ideally, be used to allow the staff to work at an easier pace (much needed after a period of extreme activity), for teaching and for tidying and checking equipment cupboards.

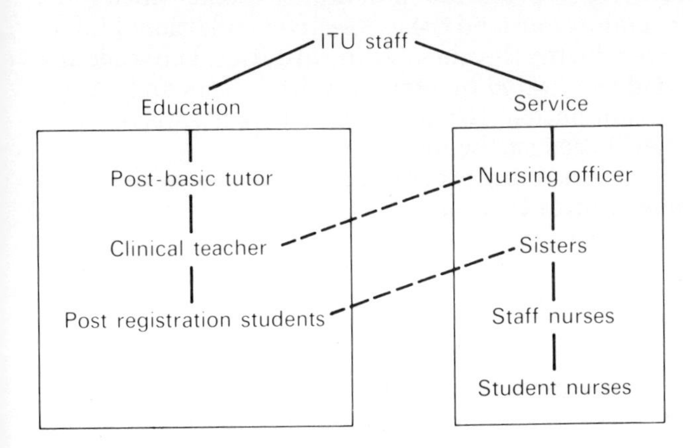

Fig. 8.1 Staffing structure.

Training

A commitment, by the senior nursing staff, to teaching and training is essential and can be considered in relation to four distinct groups of staff.

1. *The trained intensive therapy staff nurse* needs, primarily, to gain administrative experience. She should therefore take responsibility for running the unit, initially under the guidance of a sister and then, later, have sole charge on selected shifts. Time must be put aside for her to have regular instruction, both formal and informal.

2. *The untrained intensive therapy nurse* works on a unit to gain insight, perhaps, before undertaking a post-registration course, or to widen her experience. These nurses require an orientation programme to the unit during which they can be taught the essential nursing care procedures. This is followed by frequent tutorials and practical instruction. At first they should be put to work with a competent nurse, gradually taking on full responsibility for 'total patient care'.

3. *The student nurse* requires a form of instruction similar to that of the inexperienced staff nurse. Preferably, the allocation to a unit

should be during the final year of training when the experience is more meaningful.

4. *The post-registration student* attends a 26-week course for either State Registered or State Enrolled nurses (Joint Board of Clinical Nursing Studies Course 100 or 115). The syllabus for both of these courses outlines a number of educational objectives together with the skills and knowledge the nurse must attain to achieve them. The content of the lectures, tutorials and practical sessions, which total some 28 days, are planned around these objectives. Additional informal teaching is given during the nurse's clinical duties. The student's theoretical knowledge is tested by regular written tests and a final written and oral examination. Her practical ability is assessed continually during her duties on the unit.

To co-ordinate such a training programme it is necessary to have a tutor and full-time clinical teacher.

Nursing responsibilities

Nursing officers

The nursing officer has complete administrative charge and, depending on the size of the unit, may be wholly committed to the ITU or, with smaller units (less than six beds), the duties may be linked with another area. One of her main priorities is to maintain the number and quality of the nursing establishment in the unit because a great deal of stress is avoided if staffing levels are good. This, however, can at times be an extremely difficult and frustrating task. The nursing coverage of the unit has to be well planned and includes the off-duty rota and allocation of holidays. She is responsible for the selection of all grades of nursing staff to work in the unit—if not solely, then as one of an interviewing panel.

Another responsibility is to guarantee that safe nursing practices and an established standard of nursing care are constantly maintained. To achieve this a procedure manual, compiled and up-dated by the nursing officer and the sisters, is essential. In addition, the exact extent of the nurse's duties must be defined to avoid confusion between nursing and medical responsibilities. This includes, particularly, procedures such as intravenous injections, venepunctures and defibrillation. If nurses are to carry these out, then it is the nursing officer's responsibility to ensure that formal instruction, assessment and a record of competence have been made before a nurse is allowed to perform them.

The nursing officer must be involved with the post-registration course, participating in the assessment of the students' practical abilities and theoretical knowledge. She should also be very much concerned with staff welfare and at all times must be prepared to give full support and guidance to the staff.

Sisters

Ths sisters have responsibility for the day-to-day management of the unit, the teaching of staff and ensuring the provision of adequate supplies of equipment.

The major part of their work is concerned with supervision of patient care, making sure that the appropriate standard of nursing care is maintained. To organize this properly they must be aware of the individual staff nurse's capabilities and appreciate when a particular nurse requires help. In addition, they must keep the medical staff informed of relevant changes in a patient's condition and be responsible for talking to and informing relatives.

Teaching is another important aspect of their work. This involves the planning and institution of orientation and teaching programmes. Sisters are also concerned with staff morale and counselling, and for submitting regular reports on the progress of each nurse.

Organizing and maintaining stocks of equipment is another of their duties and, at the beginning of each shift, checks should be made of the equipment for emergency use, such as the resuscitation and intubation trolley. Safe use of equipment is extremely important and the sisters must ensure that the nurses know how to operate equipment safely.

Staff nurses

The staff nurses are responsible for carrying out the bedside care of the patient.

Occasionally nurses, especially new staff, may become overwhelmed by the demands of intensive care and will need help in organizing their patient care. Whilst guidelines are helpful, this is largely a subjective matter and each nurse will have her own method of planning her duties. A useful regimen is to start from the patient's head and then progress in a systematic fashion, but, because of the risks of transferring infection, always to carry out the 'clean' procedures first.

When teaching the nurse to record the various observations that she has to make, it is important to indicate the possible sources of artefacts. For instance, an arterial line may require 'flushing' before the blood pressure is measured, or the ventilator circuit checked before respiratory observations are recorded.

Organization of patient care

The organization of care must be standardized. It includes the provision of necessary equipment at each bed area, defining the routine nursing procedures that all patients are to receive and standardizing the methods of recording and charting observations.

Preparation of the bed area

The objective is to prepare the individual bed areas with the necessary equipment to make each one self-sufficient. A check list (Table 8.1) ensures that no items are omitted. All the apparatus must be tested to ensure that it is working correctly, and rechecked when an admission is expected. Each bed area must be maintained in readiness for immediate use.

After a patient has been discharged from the unit or has died, the entire bed area has to be stripped and cleaned and then refurbished.

Routine nursing procedures

These can be divided into the general duties to be maintained consistently by each shift and the specific procedures for which each shift is responsible.

On each shift the duties include:

1. Two-hourly attention to pressure sites, turning and repositioning the patient.
2. Two-hourly oral hygiene.
3. Two-hourly eye care if applicable.
4. Making appropriate observations and recording them.
5. Hourly measurement of fluid intake
6. Measurement of urine volume (hourly on catheterized patients) and other fluid losses.
7. Six-hourly aseptic catheter toilet when required.
8. Wound dressings as appropriate.
9. Restocking the bed area with syringes, needles, eye care and mouth care packs, etc.
10. Writing in the Kardex a summary of the patient's condition and events that have occurred during the shift.

The night shift duties include:

1. The blanket bath, when the bed linen is changed completely.
2. Collection of specimens; for example, sputum, blood and urine.
3. Changing the tracheal suction bottle and tubing.
4. Changing the urinary drainage system of catheterized patients.
5. Routine urine testing.

The morning shift duties include changing:

1. The oxygen mask or nasal spectacles together with the tubing and humidifier.
2. The respiratory circuit tubing, connections and humidifier container. This task may be allocated to a technician but the nurse needs to supervise it.
3. The material tape anchoring an endotracheal or tracheostomy tube.

Table 8.1 Check list for preparing a bed area (Middlesex Hospital)

Rail	
Blease air oxygen flow meter mixer	
Ventilator and humidifier (ready for use) + tubing support	
Suction unit: connect bottles for low suction, suction tubing	
Y connection for suction tubing	
Disposable catheters and Yankauer sucker in holder	
Bowl holder + 20 cm sterile bowl	
Vickers 0_2 gauge with mount for Green 0_2 tubing	
Oscillometer, blood pressure cuff and stethoscope	
Disposable gloves	
Paper masks	
Two thermometer holders (one rectal and one oral)	
Waters' canister	
Case note holder	
Shelving	
Top:	Catheter mount for endotracheal tube, swivel and 15 mm connectors Mount for Waters' canister to anaesthetic facemask + facemask airway Green 0_2 tubing + Hudson mask 1-litre bottle of sterile distilled water
Middle:	*Electrode tray*: Disposable razor and blades, electrodes, conductive gel, gauze swabs, chlorhexidine in spirit *Mouth tray*: CSSD oral hygiene packs, mouthwash tablets, tube of lanolin, bicarbonate of soda *Eye care tray*: CSSD packs, hypromellose eye drops, normal saline
bottom:	Incontinence pads Towels *Tray*: Savlon sachets, disposable flannels, hair comb, talcum powder, silicone cream
Working surface	
Tray 1:	Gauze swabs, endotracheal tube tape, safety pins, elastic bands, drawing pins, torch, additive labels, assorted plasters
Tray 2:	Needles, disposable needle container, 1 box of injection swabs (Sterets), three-way taps, occlusive sterile bungs (cap male – female Luer), 1 box of water for injection, 1 box of sodium chloride, 1 box of sodium citrate, 1 box of potassium chloride
Syringe dispenser	
Re-stock	
Charts	
Fluid balance	
General observation	

4. All the intravenous administration sets and the dressing of the puncture sites of the cannulae.
5. Chest drainage bottles and tubing.
6. Drainage bags and their tubing attached to collect fluid losses other than urine.

The afternoon shift is responsible for continuing the routine care of the patient but not specifically for changing any equipment.

At times it will be impossible, because of a changing situation, for a nurse to complete the duties allotted to the particular shift. This is of no consequence provided that the details of any omissions are communicated to the nurse taking over the patient for the next shift.

Recording and charting observations

The observation charts give a detailed record of the patient's condition and treatment up to any given moment in time. From these details important clinical decisions are made, and charting is therefore one of the important ways in which a nurse transmits information.

The number and frequency of observations are dictated by the patient's clinical condition; the nurse must be aware that in making them she may disturb the patient and therefore they should be performed as discreetly as possible. Each patient requires a minimum number of observations: hourly pulse rate, respiratory rate, blood pressure and temperature. In addition, regular records need to be kept of fluid intake and output.

ITU charts differ from ward charts because they have to accommodate a far greater number of observations. Clarity is essential and is best achieved by having a small number of separate charts with the same time span based on the 24 hour clock.

Charts required

Certain information has to be recorded about every patient; therefore, there are a number of routine charts with additional charts for special purposes. The basic charts are for general observations, fluid balance and prescription of treatment. Additional charts are required for neurological observation and for peritoneal dialysis. Details of the peritoneal dialysis chart are discussed in Chapter 22.

The general observation chart (Fig. 8.2) displays a number of physiological variables recorded graphically and alphanumerically. The use of different colours for different variables helps to avoid confusion.

The fluid balance chart (Fig. 8.3) has a number of columns on both the 'intake' and the 'output' side to provide space for the many routes of fluid administration and fluid loss. Volumes are charted hourly together with a progressive, cumulative, total. The overall state of balance is calculated at 12 and 24 hour intervals. A small electronic calculator is invaluable for performing the additions and subtractions and reduces the number of arithmetic errors. Double checking of fluid balance charts by a second nurse is essential.

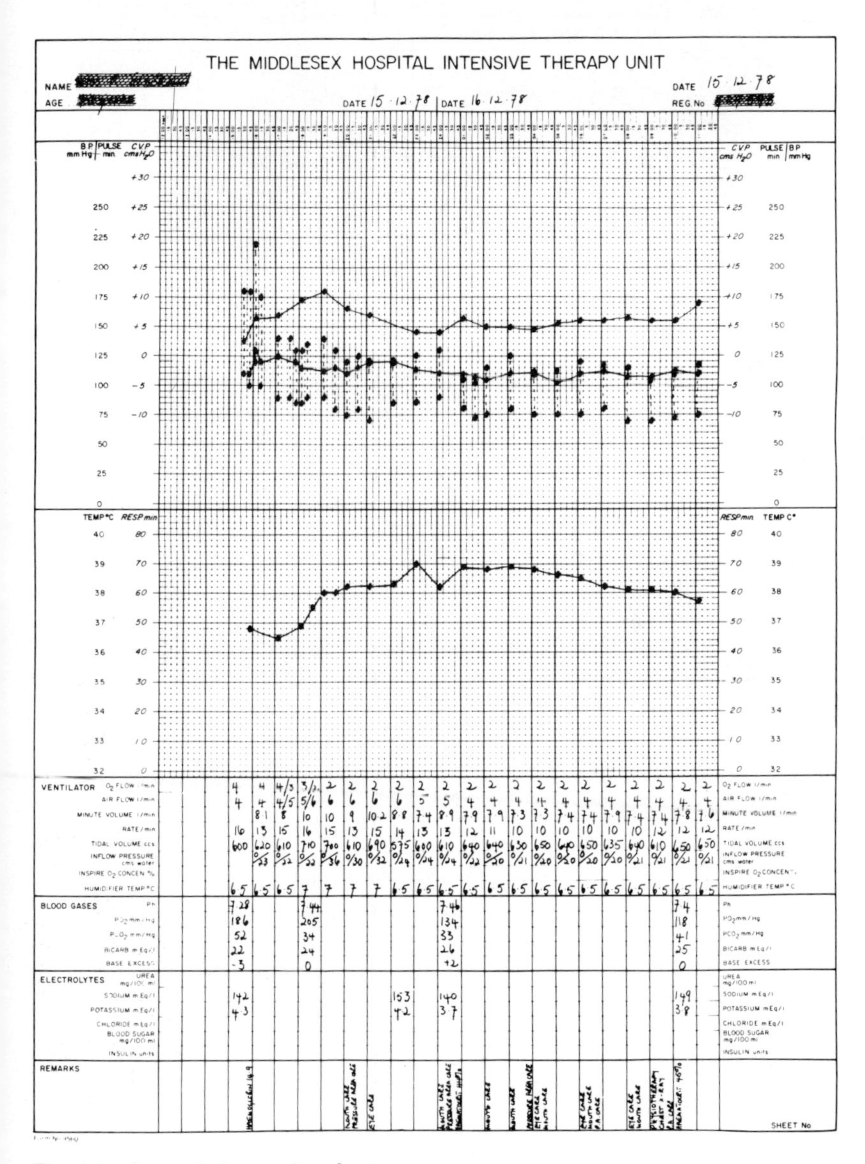

Fig. 8.2 General observation chart.

THE MIDDLESEX HOSPITAL INTENSIVE THERAPY UNIT

FLUID BALANCE CHART

NAME .... DATE FROM 16·12 TO 17·12

AGE .... REG. No ....

TIME	INPUT: N/SALINE 5% DEX SAMPLE							OUTPUT					
	Oral/NG	Intravenous 1	Intravenous 2	Intravenous 3	Additives	C.V.P. Line	Input Past Hour	NG/Tube	Urine	MIDLINE INCISION Drain	CORRUGATED Drain	Output Past Hour	Cumulative Balance
13·00	50 / 50	42 / 42	42 / 42	42 / 42	60u INSULIN (2)				55 / 55	100 / 100	15 / 15		
14·00		42 / 84	42 / 84	42 / 84	100 / 100	FLAGYL			100 / 155	200 / 300			
15·00		42 / 126	42 / 126	42 / 126					35 / 190	50+ / 350			
16·00		42 / 168	42 / 168	42 / 168				8 / 8	30 / 220	30 / 380	30 / 45		
17·00		42 / 210	42 / 210	42 / 210					55 / 275	150 / 530			
18·00	10 / 60	42 / 252	42 / 252	42 / 252					35 / 310	80 / 610			
19·00		42 / 294	42 / 294	42 / 294					50 / 360	160 / 770			
20·00		42 / 336	42 / 336	42 / 336				13 / 21	35 / 395	100 / 870	20 / 65		
21·00		42 / 378	42 / 378	42 / 378					65 / 460	150 / 1020			
22·00	15 / 75	42 / 420	42 / 420	42 / 420				14 / 35	20 / 480	175 / 1195	20 / 85		
23·00		42 / 462	42 / 462	42 / 462					19 / 499	150 / 1345			
24·00		38 / 500	42 / 504	38 / 500					40 / 539	125 / 1470			
12 HOUR TOTAL	75	500	504	500	100		1679	35	539	1470+	85		2129+
01·00		42 / 42	42 / 42	42 / 42	60u INSULIN (2)				47 / 47	100 / 100			
02·00		42 / 84	42 / 84	42 / 84				0 / 0	30 / 77	250 / 350			
03·00		70 / 154	42 / 126	42 / 126	100 / 100	FLAGYL			20 / 97	130 / 480			
04·00		70 / 224	42 / 168	42 / 168					30 / 127				
05·00	10 / 10	70 / 294	42 / 210	42 / 210					40 / 167				
06·00		70 / 364	42 / 252	42 / 252				1 / 1	60 / 227	100 / 580	25 / 25		
07·00		70 / 434	42 / 294	42 / 294					10 / 237	175 / 755			
08·00	10 / 20	70 / 504	42 / 336	42 / 336					20 / 257				
09·00	30 / 50	50 / 554	42 / 378	42 / 378					45 / 302	200 / 955			
10·00		50 / 604	42 / 420	42 / 420				3 / 4	20 / 322	200 / 1155	25 / 50		
11·00		50 / 654	42 / 462	42 / 462					12 / 334	280 / 1435			
12·00		50 / 704	42 / 504	42 / 504					25 / 359	100 / 1535			
12 HOUR TOTAL	50	704	504	504	100			4	359	1535	50		
24 HOUR TOTAL	125	1204	1008	1004	200		3541	39	898	3005+	135		4077+

URINE ANALYSIS

Time 06·00
S.G. 1010
pH 5
Sugar NEG
Acetone NEG
Albumin NEG
Blood SMALL
Bilirubin LARGE
Urobilinogen 12

24 HOUR INPUT = 3541

OUTPUT = 4077+

BALANCE = −536

FORM 123 (FIRST REVISION) Sheet No ....

Fig. 8.3 Fluid balance chart.

The prescription chart (Fig. 8.4) has to cater for a large and unpredictable number of drugs and intravenous fluids. It must have sufficient space for the writing and recording of prescriptions, together with the time of administration and signatures of the two nurses who check the prescription. A new chart should be prepared each day to avoid confusion.

Form No. M 46 (FIRST REVISION)

THE MIDDLESEX HOSPITAL INTENSIVE THERAPY UNIT
TREATMENT CARD

DRUG HYPERSENSITIVITIES
1 PENICILLIN 3 ....
2 .... 4 ....

SURNAME [illegible] REG. NO. [illegible]
FIRST NAMES [illegible] DATE OF BIRTH [illegible]

DATE	DRUG	DOSE & FREQUENCY OF ADMINISTRATION	ROUTE	DOCTOR'S SIGNATURE	FLUID REGIME	DOCTOR'S SIGNATURE
1.3.79	GENTAMICIN	80mg 12·20·04	I.V.		500 mls 50% DEXTROSE 12—24 + 40units SOLUBLE INSULIN 24—12	
1.3.79	OMNOPON	5-10mg. 2 hourly p.r.n.	I.V.		500 mls INTRALIPID 10% 12—24 24—12	
1.3.79	CIMETIDINE	200mg 12·18·24·06	I.V.		500 mls. SYNTHAMIN 14 12—24 + 30 mmol KCL 24—12	
					500 mls 5% DEXTROSE to read C.V.P.	
					SHEET No.......	

Fig. 8.4 Prescription chart.

The neurological observation chart (Fig. 8.5) must provide a correct and easily understandable account of the neurological state of a patient. Different nurses will make the observations on the same patient and conformity of description is essential. The Glasgow Coma Scale (described in Chapter 25) presents the necessary information without resorting to vague descriptive terms.

It is important that all observations are recorded clearly and neatly and that, if a colour coded system is used, this is not varied because confusion may arise. Untidy charts are dangerous.

Many charts, documents and reports concerning the patient accumulate during his stay in the unit. For convenience and ease of retrieval it is useful to have a loose-leaf ring folder in which the medical notes, prescription charts and results can be filed. On discharge of the patient to the ward the contents of this folder are transferred to the case notes and, for the convenience of the ward staff, ward observation charts are completed to cover the previous 24 hours.

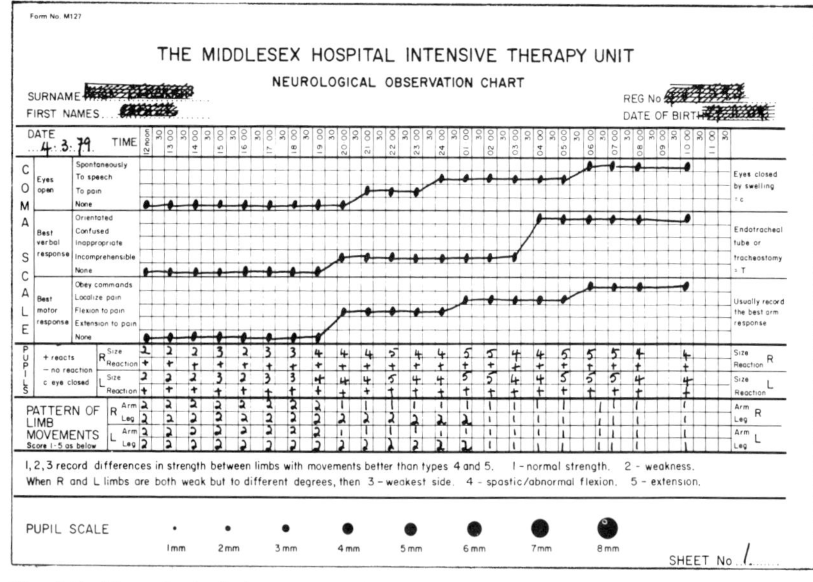
Form No. M127

THE MIDDLESEX HOSPITAL INTENSIVE THERAPY UNIT

NEUROLOGICAL OBSERVATION CHART

SURNAME .... REG No ....

FIRST NAMES .... DATE OF BIRTH ....

DATE 4.3.79 TIME 12 noon, 30, 13 00, 30, 14 00, 30, 15 00, 30, 16 00, 30, 17 00, 30, 18 00, 30, 19 00, 30, 20 00, 30, 21 00, 30, 22 00, 30, 23 00, 30, 24 00, 30, 01 00, 30, 02 00, 30, 03 00, 30, 04 00, 30, 05 00, 30, 06 00, 30, 07 00, 30, 08 00, 30, 09 00, 30, 10 00, 30, 11 00, 30

COMA SCALE

Eyes open: Spontaneously / To speech / To pain / None — Eyes closed by swelling = C

Best verbal response: Orientated / Confused / Inappropriate / Incomprehensible / None — Endotracheal tube or tracheostomy = T

Best motor response: Obey commands / Localize pain / Flexion to pain / Extension to pain / None — Usually record the best arm response

PUPILS: + reacts, − no reaction, c eye closed — R Size / Reaction; L Size / Reaction

PATTERN OF LIMB MOVEMENTS Score 1-5 as below — R Arm / Leg; L Arm / Leg

1, 2, 3 record differences in strength between limbs with movements better than types 4 and 5. 1 - normal strength. 2 - weakness. When R and L limbs are both weak but to different degrees, then 3 - weakest side. 4 - spastic/abnormal flexion. 5 - extension.

PUPIL SCALE 1mm 2mm 3mm 4mm 5mm 6mm 7mm 8mm

SHEET No. 1

Fig. 8.5 Neurological observation chart.

Stress of intensive therapy

In recent years much has been written about the stresses imposed by an ITU on patients, their relatives and the staff. Whilst undoubtedly of great consequence, it is important to keep it in perspective for ITUs are by no means the only areas in hospitals that generate stressful situations. The occurrence of such problems can be readily reduced by a sensitive and considerate approach by the nursing staff to the patient and their relatives, and from the nursing officer and sisters to the other nurses.

The patient

It must always be assumed that seemingly unconscious patients can hear and understand. The patient must always be greeted by name, given an explanation of every procedure before it takes place, reassured about treatment and progress, and given constant sensory stimulation by general conversation from the nurse and relatives when they visit. Sometimes playing a radio may help, provided the patient's tastes in listening have been previously established.

The conscious patient of course requires the same explanations and reassurance. Often the communication barrier of an endotracheal or tracheostomy tube needs to be overcome. The inability to speak can be extremely frustrating and frightening for a patient. Repeated assurance that this is only a temporary measure is necessary, and every effort must be made to make communication as easy as possible. Various methods can be used, such as sign language, writing or supplying an alphabet to which the patient can point. Normal orientation is helped by the presence of a clock and a calendar that the patient can see from his bed. The use of radios, tape recorders, talking books and even television should be encouraged to increase the patients's awareness of the 'real world'.

Nursing routines should be arranged to provide adequate periods of rest and sleep for the patient. Sleep deprivation produces irritability, depression, delirium, hallucinations and disorientation. These manifestations are commonly referred to as the 'white wall or ITU syndrome' and have all been attributed to the environment of an ITU where constant noise, light and activity are considered normal and necessary. Sleep deprivation must be diminished to an absolute minimum. It is important to distinguish between day and night, by dimming the main lights at night, and as far as possible to maintain the normal pattern of sleep. Observations and treatments should, where possible, be reduced during the night to allow the patient to have the maximum amount of uninterrupted rest.

The relatives

Relatives and friends visiting patients in an ITU are naturally extremely anxious. A sympathetic and understanding approach by both medical and nursing staff is essential to allay some of their anxieties. They need to be kept fully informed of the patient's condition and told truthfully the expected course of events in terms that they can easily understand. This has to include a simple explanation of the equipment, why it is being used and what is hoped it will achieve. People in an anxious state have limited powers of concentration and often forget what they have been told so that repeated explanations are necessary; to avoid misinterpretation, staff talking to relatives must know what has been said previously, or will be said by other members of staff, since variations of terminology can lead to unfortunate misunderstandings.

At their first visit, relatives must be given a detailed explanation before they actually enter the unit. The activities of an ITU are strange and foreign to the majority of people. Unrestricted visiting should be the unit's policy, with the sisters using discretion as to who visits and for how long. A great deal of comfort and encouragement may be gained by patients when their relatives are with them, although they must never be made to feel obliged to stay constantly. It should be conveyed to relatives that telephone enquiries are not regarded as a nuisance, and when they are made they must be answered courteously, carefully and with appropriate discretion.

A unit must provide a comfortable waiting-room and overnight accommodation for relatives. When relatives stay at the hospital they may need sedation in order to get a good night's sleep. Encouraging them to go out for short walks or perhaps a meal may temporarily help to relieve the burden of their anxieties.

For patients who are to be admitted electively after surgery, anxiety and apprehension can often be reduced, for both the patient and their relatives, if they are allowed to visit the unit beforehand. A brief explanatory talk and the opportunity to meet some of the staff does a great deal to instil confidence.

The nurse

Intensive therapy nursing imposes physical, mental and emotional strains on the nurse, for she carries many responsibilities and will inevitably feel some emotional involvement with the patient and relatives.

Some of these strains are reduced by a cheerful and less formal working atmosphere. It is essential that easy communication amongst the staff is maintained. Delegating one sister to be responsible for a particular group of nurses makes it easy for them to identify with a senior member of the nursing staff and encourages counselling. Regular unit meetings, where everyone can congregate and talk freely, are also of benefit.

Nurses do become attached to their patient and involved with the family. This involvement is heightened in an ITU by the necessity of having one nurse looking after one patient, which naturally produces a close relationship. Some nurses are able to cope well with these emotional demands whilst others find them stressful. To a certain extent this situation can be relieved by allocating a different nurse each day to one patient.

Additional stress can be avoided if the medical organization includes having a doctor present in the unit throughout the 24 hours. This means that nurses are never left in the position of having to make decisions or take action beyond their capabilities while waiting for the medical staff to arrive.

The morale of a unit depends on the professional relationships of the medical and nursing personnel. The success of this relies largely on clear guidelines on individual responsibility, a regard for each other's professional skills, easy communication and an acceptance of colleagues' views—the essence of team work.

9

Practical procedures

In this chapter the general aspects of practical nursing care are considered. The procedures relating to total patient care and specific systems that are not included in other chapters are described. This is followed by the techniques for controlling body temperature and the administration of intravenous fluids and drugs.

Total patient care

Skin

Care is required to ensure the comfort of the patient, maintain hygiene, prevent friction or pressure complications and protect the skin from irritating discharges. It involves blanket bathing, protection of the skin from friction or pressure and the use of barrier preparations.

Blanket bathing
A blanket bath is needed each day and at the same time the nurse also attends to the patient's personal appearance (nails, hair, shaving). Additional washes are necessary if the patient is perspiring or incontinent. The skin, particularly in the groins and axillae, must be thoroughly dried afterwards to discourage the development of sore areas. If the skin is too dry, an emulsifying ointment may help.

Protection from friction or pressure
In the seriously ill patient many factors such as immobility, incontinence, hypotension and long periods spent on hard operating tables predispose to the breakdown of the skin. Extra risks are presented in paraplegic patients because of the loss of skin sensation and circulatory control.

Friction is generated by almost any movement of the patient and is therefore greater if the patient is restless. It is increased in all instances if the bed linen is wet.

Prevention. Dry bed linen is essential, and when the patient is moved he must always be lifted and never pulled. In sitting positions, sliding movements can be avoided by placing a bolster at the patient's feet or slightly elevating the foot of the bed.

Pressure on vulnerable areas such as the shoulders, spine, buttocks and heels is inevitable. These sites are well recognized by nurses and none of them must be neglected.

Prevention. Regular, two-hourly, turning relieves pressure in most instances; if a patient's skin marks easily, hourly changes of position may be necessary. At least two nurses are needed to turn and reposition a patient. Before starting, it is important to ensure that apparatus connected to the patient is adjusted so that it is not inadvertently detached and does not pull on the skin. If the patient is intubated, one nurse should concentrate solely on positioning the head and neck. Careful handling of the limbs is necessary to avoid unsupported movements. The patient must not be left lying on apparatus, and pillows are used to support the body and ease pressure between the legs in lateral positions. The judicious use of sandbags or plaster of Paris splints can counteract the development of foot drop and contractures of the Achilles tendon. During turning, the performance of passive limb movements prevents joint stiffness, contractures and circulatory complications.

Each time the patient is turned and repositioned skin hygiene to the pressure sites is maintained and is supplemented by gentle massage using a light dusting of talcum powder or, if the skin is dry, a small amount of moisture cream. Vigorous rubbing with soap and water is harmful because it can damage and remove natural oils from the skin. If red pressure areas do appear, for example, on the buttocks, pressure is relieved by nursing the patient in the lateral positions until the redness has disappeared.

Methods of relieving pressure

There are three types of aids to relieve pressure.

1. Ripple or bubble pad mattresses alternate areas of pressure contact by cyclical inflation and deflation of the sections or cells.

2. Synthetic gel cushions alleviate pressure by suspension, and when the patient changes position they recover their original shape.

3. Sheepskin pads and heel bootees reduce friction but are ineffective if they become wet. Heel bootees must not be fastened too tightly or they will obstruct venous return from the feet.

All these devices, though helpful, are only aids; they are not substitutes for the regular turning and repositioning of the patient.

A variety of special beds are available for counteracting pressure but none of them is suitable for use in an ITU because of the problems they pose during resuscitation.

Barrier preparations
These are used to prevent breakdown of the skin from irritating discharges. They consist of silicone, which prevents moisture from getting to the skin, and are used in the presence of urinary or faecal incontinence. Stomahesive and Orabase paste are ideal, non-sensitizing, preparations to protect the skin around pancreatic, gastric and biliary drains or fistulae, where the fluids may digest the skin. Stomahesive is supplied in squares which mould to the skin contours. The square is prepared by cutting a central hole to fit around the drain or fistula, leaving as little skin exposed as possible. It provides a secure base onto which a collecting bag can be attached. Orabase paste can be used alone or in conjunction with Stomahesive. It is used to prevent sutures becoming embedded in the Stomahesive, to form a seal around the base of a fistula or drain and to fill any gaps the Stomahesive has not covered.

Eyes

If the eyes are not protected properly they may become infected or damaged. This is most likely to happen when the blink reflex is lost as occurs in coma, or after neuromuscular blocking drugs. The presence of corneal oedema aggravates the situation as does the drying effect of oxygen that is blown across the face.

The eyes need to be bathed aseptically every two hours with swabs soaked in normal saline and artificial tears (hypromellose) instilled. If the eyes remain open the lids should be closed with strips of micropore tape. Eye pads are not used because if the patient blinks the cornea may be scratched. Each time eye care is carried out the eyes are inspected for signs of inflammation or a discharge. If either is present a swab is sent for culture and the appropriate antibiotic drops or ointment is included in the care.

Nares

When a patient is incapable of blowing his nose, cleaning is required to remove secretions. This is particularly so when one of the nasal passages is used for the insertion of an endotracheal or nasogastric tube. Careful anchorage of either is essential to prevent pulling the skin, pressure can be relieved by placing small pieces of gauze between the tube and the skin.

Each nostril is gently cleaned, as required, using cotton wool buds soaked in normal saline. It is not done in patients with head injuries or cerebrospinal fluid leakage because of the danger of infection or increasing the amount of drainage. In these instances any discharge is simply wiped away.

Ears

Washing the ears at the time of the blanket bath is sufficient unless a discharge, blood or cerebrospinal fluid is visible in the external meatus. A discharge is commonly the result of local infection and is treated with antibiotic drops. Bleeding or cerebrospinal fluid drainage are complications of head injury and the aims of care are to keep the ears clean by dry mopping. The discharge is irritating if it remains on the skin.

When a patient is nursed in the lateral positions it is important that the ears lie flat against the pillow to avoid discomfort and pressure complications. It is also important to ensure that the tubing or elastic of either nasal spectacles or an oxygen mask are not pulled tightly over the top of the ears.

Gastrointestinal tract

Nasogastric tubes (Ryle's)

These are passed into the stomach for the purpose of feeding or aspiration. They are often difficult to pass in intubated patients and frequently need to be introduced under direct vision using a laryngoscope. Once passed, their position is confirmed by standard methods.

When used for aspiration, suction is applied at least hourly with a syringe or, alternatively, the tube is connected to a disposable collecting bag and allowed to drain freely. Accurate records of the volumes aspirated must be charted and incorporated into the patient's fluid balance. The frequency of aspiration is reduced as the volume of gastric aspirate decreases but failure to aspirate any fluid should prompt the nurse to check the position of the tube.

Mouth

Several problems can develop if adequate mouth care is not given. Neglect leads to ulceration, fungal infections and parotitis. Many patients mouth breathe, some have reduced salivary secretions whilst others have increased flow, stimulated by the presence of an oral endotracheal tube.

To keep the mouth clean and moist two-hourly oral hygiene is required. This is not an aseptic procedure but must be performed as a 'socially clean' one to avoid introducing infection. Excess saliva is removed by suction and various solutions (thymol, glycerine and lemon, and sodium bicarbonate) are used to swab the mouth. Lanolin or white petroleum jelly is applied to the lips and corners of the mouth to prevent drying and cracking.

When an oral endotracheal tube or Guedal airway is *in situ*, oral hygiene is more difficult. Compressible sponge swabs make access easier. A Guedel airway needs to be changed every 12 hours and four-hourly if there are a lot of secretions. Pressure on the lips or corners of the mouth from an endotracheal tube can be eliminated by supporting the tube away from these areas using gauze or sponge material.

A white coating in the mouth is often a sign of *Candida albicans* infection for which local nystatin preparations are effective. The diagnosis should be confirmed by taking a swab for culture.

Gastrostomy or jejunostomy

Either of these may be fashioned as a means of aspirating gastric contents or as a method of feeding. The gastrostomy or jejunostomy catheter is always sealed with a spigot and never left to drain freely because large volumes of intestinal fluid can be lost, particularly if the patient is in a lateral position. Aspiration is carried out intermittently, and the volume aspirated accurately measured.

When a gastrostomy or jejunostomy is used for feeding, the same principles apply as for a nasogastric tube. Feeding is started gradually, using a funnel so that the feeds run in by gravity. The insertion site of the catheter is observed for regurgitation of fluid, and if this occurs the rate of administration is decreased. It is protected by a sterile dressing which is renewed at least daily.

Bowel

Damage to the rectal mucosa can be produced when measuring rectal temperature. Gentle insertion of either an electronic probe or mercury thermometer is essential. If handled carelessly, a mercury thermometer can break in the rectum.

Immobility often leads to constipation and flatulence. Regular bowel function is aided by the use of enemas, suppositories or laxatives. Flatus can be relieved by passing a rectal catheter. Some patients have diarrhoea, which may be a symptom of their illness, due to faecal impaction or associated with nasogastric feeding. The insertion of a rectal catheter attached to a disposable drainage bag helps to reduce faecal incontinence and prevents skin excoriation.

Genitourinary system

Urethral catheterization permits accurate and continuous measurement of urinary output. It is necessary in all patients where fluid balance is critical. In some male patients, especially the elderly because of prostatic enlargement, it may be preferable to avoid catheterization and to use, instead, an external latex rubber or plastic sheath.

Unless catheters are properly managed, urinary tract infections occur. Catheter care must be observed by attention to:

1. Strict asepsis during insertion.
2. Maintenance of a closed drainage system—which is changed aseptically daily, at which time specimens of urine are taken for culture and routine testing.
3. Anchoring the catheter securely.
4. Performing six-hourly catheter toilet to reduce the incidence of ascending urinary infection.

Type of catheter

The most frequently used self-retaining catheter is a Foley catheter which has an inflatable balloon near its tip, allowing the catheter to be retained in the bladder. Each is clearly labelled with the balloon volume and they are made of latex or silicone rubber, or polyvinylchloride.

Latex rubber catheters are suitable for short-term use, up to seven days. They are, however, irritant to the lining of the urethra and predispose to encrustation and infection, and should be changed after this time.

Polyvinylchloride catheters can be left in place for up to four weeks since they are less irritant to the urethra.

Silicone rubber catheters are considerably more expensive than the other types and their use is generally reserved for long-term catheterization. They are less irritant and replacement every two months is a safe rule of practice.

Control of body temperature

Body temperature is regulated by a sensitive control mechanism, with a central regulating centre in the hypothalamus. Core temperature is normally maintained within narrow limits and when there is a tendency for it to rise, vasodilatation and sweating occur and heat loss is increased. Conversely, when the body temperature falls, vasoconstriction occurs and preserves body heat. The temperature-regulating mechanism can be altered by certain drugs (such as the phenothiazines which produce hypothermia) or disturbed by infection and intracranial pathology when hyperthermia occurs. With infection, as body temperature rises there is a paradoxical vasoconstriction and increased shivering (rigor). This prevents heat loss and increases heat production, leading to a rapid rise in temperature.

Active measures become necessary to reduce body temperature when it rises above 39°C and to increase it when it falls below 33°C. The main concern in hypothermia is the occurrence of ventricular dysrhythmias. Hyperthermia produces a marked increase in metabolic rate and oxygen demands, and in children can cause febrile convulsions.

Techniques for reducing temperature

Tepid sponging lowers the temperature by evaporation of water from the skin. The body is sponged with cool water (approximately 27°C). Cold compresses or ice bags placed in the groins and axillae may be useful supplements. The compresses need to be changed regularly and the skin protected against ice burns by putting each bag in a pillow case. The body temperature is measured at the beginning of sponging and 10 minutes after completion of the procedure, which should take no longer than 15–20 minutes to complete. If tepid sponging proves ineffective then the skin may be sponged with a solution of alcohol.

Continuous cooling can be achieved by reducing the environmental temperature, nursing the patient between wet sheets, using cold compresses or ice bags or creating a flow of cold air across the patient with a fan. In some cases a combination of these methods may be required.

Some patients find cooling procedures distressing and will need reassurance; others find them relaxing and refreshing.

Drugs can be used to reduce body temperature. Their use should, however, not replace aggressive nursing methods. Aspirin lowers body temperature by a direct action on the temperature-regulating centre and can be given conveniently by suppository. Chlorpromazine causes vasodilatation and lowers body temperature by increasing heat loss.

Technique for increasing temperature

Rewarming is carried out slowly at a room temperature of 25–32°C using insulation around the patient to prevent loss of heat.

Rapid rewarming is rarely necessary and the use of an electric blanket or hot water bottles may cause burns.

Insulation is achieved by covering the patient (apart from the face) with a flannelette or similar thin sheet; this is then covered by a sheet of aluminium foil ('space blanket') which is tucked tightly around the patient. Procedures that require removal of the sheets are kept to a minimum and the core temperature (rectal) is monitored continuously.

Intravenous infusions

Setting up an intravenous infusion must be done with absolute sterility to minimize the risks of local or systemic infection. Careful preparation of all the equipment is necessary and avoidance of contact with unsterile areas essential. Once the cannula is in position, the primed administration set is connected. When more than one solution is to be given at a time, a three-way tap, four-way junction tube or similar item must be connected between the catheter and the giving set. Peripheral lines can be anchored with adhesive plaster but one or two sutures are necessary to ensure firm stabilization of a central catheter. The site is covered with either a sterile gauze or a transparent dressing. The risk of infection during the infusion is reduced by:

1. Daily aseptic changing of the dressing, unless a transparent one is used, and inspection for signs of infection.
2. Setting up each solution aseptically and, when air venting is required, changing the airway with each bottle making sure that the cotton wool plug is not absent or wet since both of these are sources of contamination.
3. Changing the administration set (or sets) and any connectors daily or after completion of a plasma, blood or fat infusion.
4. Not withdrawing blood samples from the catheter.
5. Giving all intravenous drugs aseptically and preparing solutions with additives at the required time, not in advance.

The subsequent principles of care are the same irrespective of the type of solution being infused or the site of infusion. Many patients have more than one infusion in progress at a time and accurate records of each solution must be maintained with the hourly quantity infused and the running balance.

The nurse must observe the individual infusions and check that:

1. The solution is dripping satisfactorily at the prescribed rate. Burette giving sets make the hourly infusion rate easy to calculate; simply divide the volume of fluid by the number of hours over which it

is to be given. When their use is impractical, as during a blood transfusion, a spring balance helps to measure flow rates.

2. Obstruction of the line does not occur.

3. Tension on the line is avoided to prevent disconnection or pulling the cannula out of the vein.

4. The infusion is not running into the subcutaneous tissues. This is particularly relevant when sodium bicarbonate, dopamine and noradrenaline are being infused because leakage into the surrounding tissues can cause tissue necrosis.

5. There is no evidence of thrombophlebitis. At the first sign of sepsis, the infusion is discontinued, the cannula removed and blood cultures are taken. In addition, if a plastic cannula was in place, the tip is sent for culture.

The safe managment of intravenous therapy cannot be overemphasized. It requires careful checking of the prescribed solution and its expiry date, diligent aseptic practice and accurate infusion rate. In addition, before blood is transfused it is essential that the details on the bag conform with those on the haematology form. During the transfusion the patient must be observed for signs of incompatibility indicated by a rise in either the pulse rate or temperature, a rash or complaints from the patient of back pain.

Administration of intravenous drugs

This can be done by adding the drugs to the infusion bag or bottle, or to the chamber of the burette. They may also be injected directly through the 'target' site of an infusion set or through a three-way tap. Whichever entry port is used, the insertion site must be cleansed with an antiseptic and allowed to dry before the drug is injected. The risk of introducing infection is considered to be higher when drugs are given through a three-way tap because of the difficulties of cleaning the entry port; between use, this site is sealed with an occlusive sterile bung.

To avoid errors intravenous drugs should be prescribed clearly, stating:

1. The name and dose of the drug.
2. The frequency with which it can or must be given.
3. The route by which it is to be administered.
4. The solution and volume in which it is to be diluted, if required.
5. The period of time over which the drug is to be administered.

Once a drug has been added to an infusion solution or burette, a clear label giving the name of the drug and its dose should be attached to the container and removed from the burette once the administration is completed.

Drugs should ideally be added only to saline or dextrose solutions and never mixed with other infusions. To avoid chemical incompatibility it is advisable not to add more than one drug to an infusion solution, although certain combinations are known to be safe (Table 9.1). Chemical incompatibility is seldom a problem with direct injection of a drug but the drip rate needs to be increased for a few seconds to flush the drug through the cannula.

Table 9.1 Acceptable drug combinations

Antibiotics	Ampicillin Benzylpenicillin Cephalothin Cephradine Erythromycin Flucloxacillin
Inotropic agents	Adrenaline Dopamine Isoprenaline
Others	Dextrose Insulin Potassium cloride

From *A Guide to Intravenous Drug Administration*, Kensington and Chelsea and Westminster Area Health Authority (Teaching)

Automatic infusion systems

These are required when a drug in a solution has to be given by continuous intravenous infusion. The traditional method of drop counting and hand regulation of the drip set is far too time consuming and inaccurate. Various types of automatic infusion systems are now available, the most popular being volumetric pumps and drop counters (Fig. 9.1). These differ in their mode of action: a volumetric pump performs like a syringe, infusing at a rate measured in millilitres per hour; with drop counters the fluid is 'dripped' at a pre-set drop rate by a peristaltic finger pump.

In operating these devices the nurse must understand the principles of the system in use. In particular she must know the number of drops equivalent to one millilitre of the various infusion sets, for this is undoubtedly the major source of error. Most burette systems—for example, Soluset and Buretrol—give 60 drops/ml whilst some administration sets for blood and blood derivatives have a larger drop size, with 15 drops being equal to 1 ml.

When one of these devices is in use the nurse needs to make routine checks to ensure that all the connections are attached and that air has not entered the system. An alarm to detect such faults is incorporated but the nurse must not rely entirely on this, since a period of time may elapse before the alarm operates.

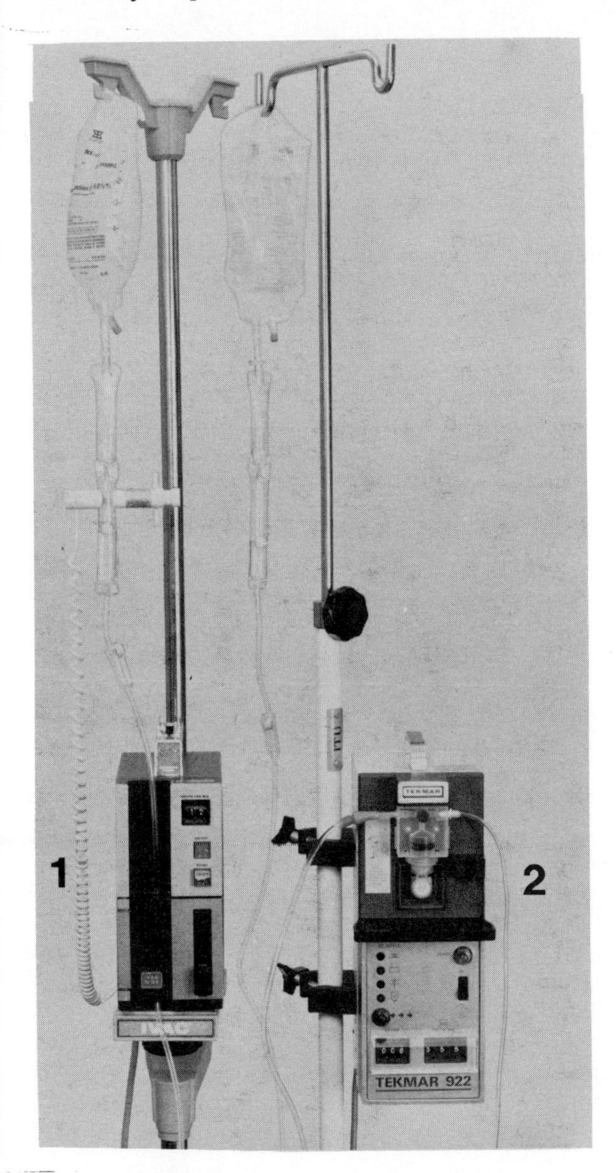

Fig. 9.1 Automatic infusion systems: 1. a drop counter (Ivac); 2. a volumetric pump (Tekmar).

10
Feeding

Full nutritional support is an essential part of the management of critically ill patients. Severe illness or injury markedly increases the rate of catabolism and produces a state of negative nitrogen balance. As a consequence, in the seriously ill both the calorie and nitrogen requirements are increased some three- or fourfold and, not surprisingly, without adequate feeding patients rapidly lose weight; loss of more than one-third of the body weight is associated with a high mortality.

The important metabolic changes are:
1. a great increase in catabolism;
2. a negative nitrogen balance;
3. depletion of carbohydrate reserves;
4. fluid and electrolyte disturbances.

Failure to control these causes:
1. hypoproteinaemia;
2. oedema;
3. increased susceptibility to infection;
4. delayed wound healing and wound dehiscence.

All of these are largely attributable, directly or indirectly, to relative protein lack.

The purpose of feeding is to replenish losses that have already occurred, to correct catabolism and, if possible, promote anabolism. These aims can be attained if sufficient calories and nitrogen are supplied. The requirements are high—4000 calories and 80 g of protein (12.8 g nitrogen*) (Table 10.1)—well above the normal demands of 2000–2500 calories and 40 g of protein (6.4 g nitrogen*).

The rate of catabolism can also be reduced by the prompt treatment of infection, control of hyperthermia (a rise of 1°C increases catabolism by 10–20 per cent) and the use of insulin and anabolic steroids.

* 1 g protein = 1/6.25 g nitrogen.

Table 10.1 Basic calorie and nitrogen requirements of specific types of patients

Clinical condition	Calories (per 24 hours)	Nitrogen (g per 24 hours)
Uncomplicated postoperative	2000–3000	10–15
Complicated postoperative Severe infections Major injuries	3500–5000	15–25
Major burns	5000	25+

Components of feeding

Calories can be supplied in the form of carbohydrate, fat or alcohol, each of which has a different calorific value: 1 g of carbohydrate = 4 calories; 1 g of fat = 9 calories; and 1 g of alcohol = 7 calories.

Protein can be given either as natural protein or in the form of amino acids. A minimum of 200 calories should be supplied for every gram of nitrogen given, to ensure that it is utilized for protein synthesis and not broken down for the provision of energy.

Water and electrolyte requirements are provided according to the principles outlined in Chapter 4.

Vitamin supplements must be given. Table 10.2 indicates their various functions.

Mineral elements are essential for maintaining certain physiological functions. Calcium, phosphorus and magnesium are constituents of bones and teeth. Sodium and chloride are major con-

Table 10.2 Functions of certain vitamins

Vitamin	Function
Thiamine (vitamin B_1)	Release of energy from carbohydrate
Riboflavine (vitamin B_2)	Utilization of energy from food
Nicotinic acid	Utilization of energy from food
Pyridoxine (vitamin B_6)	Metabolism of amino acids; formation of haemoglobin
Cyanocobalamin (vitamin B_{12})	Red cell formation
Folic acid	Red cell formation
Pantothenic acid	Release of energy from fat and carbohydrate
Biotin (vitamin H)	Metabolism of fat
Ascorbic acid (vitamin C)	Maintenance of healthy connective tissue
Vitamin K	Formation of prothrombin in the liver

stituents of extracellular fluid; potassium, magnesium and phosphorus of intracellular fluid; and iron and phosphorus are essential components of many enzymes and other proteins. These seven elements, together with sulphur which is present in a number of amino acids, are termed the major elements. The remainder, shown in Table 10.3, are referred to as trace elements.

Table 10.3 Functions of trace elements

Trace element	Function
Cobalt	Utilized in the formation of vitamin B_{12}
Copper	Associated with a number of enzymes
Chromium	Involved in the utilization of glucose
Fluorine	Associated with the structure of bones and teeth
Iodine	Essential constituent of hormones produced by the thyroid gland
Manganese	Associated with a number of enzymes
Zinc	Associated with wound healing

Methods of feeding

There are three ways of providing food: conventionally, through a nasogastric tube or intravenously.

Of all these methods eating is, of course, the ideal, but the seriously ill patient is often anorexic or nauseated. He may be unconscious, have an endotracheal tube *in situ* or be suffering from neurological disease all of which make eating difficult or impossible.

Eating

If the patient can take food then every effort must be made to encourage him to eat. Trouble should be taken to serve the patient's favourite foods, and meals need to look attractive and be given in amounts that can be tolerated. Appetite stimulants or aperitifs may be of some help but are usually disappointing.

Even with attention to these details, provision of the necessary requirements is often difficult; the patients cannot tolerate the bulk of food needed to supply sufficient calories. Drinks are a useful alternative and are made with ingredients such as glucose, fruit, milk, Complan and eggs so that additional protein, fats and vitamins are given at the same time. For those patients who are unable to tolerate milk, ice cream is an appropriate substitute. Hycal, a protein-free, low-electrolyte liquid dextrose available in different flavours, is a good source of calories but unfortunately many patients are unable to tolerate its sweetness.

When a patient can eat only small amounts of food, meals have to be supplemented by a balanced, palatable, liquid diet. Two different forms may be used, consisting of either undigested or predigested foodstuffs.

Undigested foodstuffs such as Complan and Clinifeed are both complete liquid diets containing carbohydrate, fat, protein, vitamins and minerals. These products are suitable for patients with normal digestion.

Complan is a soluble powder and each pack gives a detailed list of its constituents and instructions for dilution. If a whole day's supply is prepared at one time, it must be stored in a refrigerator. It is available in a number of different flavours and may be served hot or cold.

Clinifeed is presented in cans as a liquid, flavoured with either chocolate or vanilla. The amount of fat, protein, vitamins and minerals varies according to the preparation. It can be stored at room temperature, but once the can is opened it must be kept refrigerated and any unused fluid discarded after 24 hours. Before administration, each can should be diluted to 500 ml to reduce the risk of osmotic diarrhoea.

Predigested foodstuffs are liquid, chemically defined diets. They provide the essential nutrients in a pre-digested or elemental form: protein as amino acids, fat as triglyceride and carbohydrate as glucose; vitamins and minerals are added. This type of diet is beneficial for patients with digestive and absorptive disorders—particularly inflammatory disease of the bowel, gastrointestinal fistulae and following major bowel surgery. Absorption is completed in the upper gastrointestinal tract and the residue is small.

Elemental diets are sold as soluble powders in varying nutritional quantities and in a variety of flavours. They are prepared by dissolving an appropriate amount in the prescribed quantity of water or milk, and taste better if served well chilled. Once made, they must be stored in a refrigerator. They can also be prepared as jellies or ice lollies—an easy way of giving them to children.

Whichever type of liquid diet is used, it is better tolerated if given slowly in small quantities, 100–200 ml at a time. Larger volumes may cause nausea and vomiting. However, in spite of these precautions, it may still prove impossible to provide the total requirements. Eating has then to be supplemented with another method of feeding.

Nasogastric tube feeding

This, in general, is used in patients who, for some reason, are unable to swallow but who have normal alimentary function; for example, the unconscious or intubated patient.

Method

A feeding tube (a fine-bore Ryle's tube or similar narrow-bore tube) is passed into the stomach via the nose and its position is checked by standard methods. The tube must be firmly secured to prevent displacement or inadvertent removal by the patient or nurse. It may be anchored to the patient's nose with either adhesive plaster or a silk suture or fixed in a self-adhesive retainer attached to the patient's forehead (Fig. 10.1). Whichever method is used, cleaning the nostril and minimizing pressure from the tube are important to prevent ulceration of the skin.

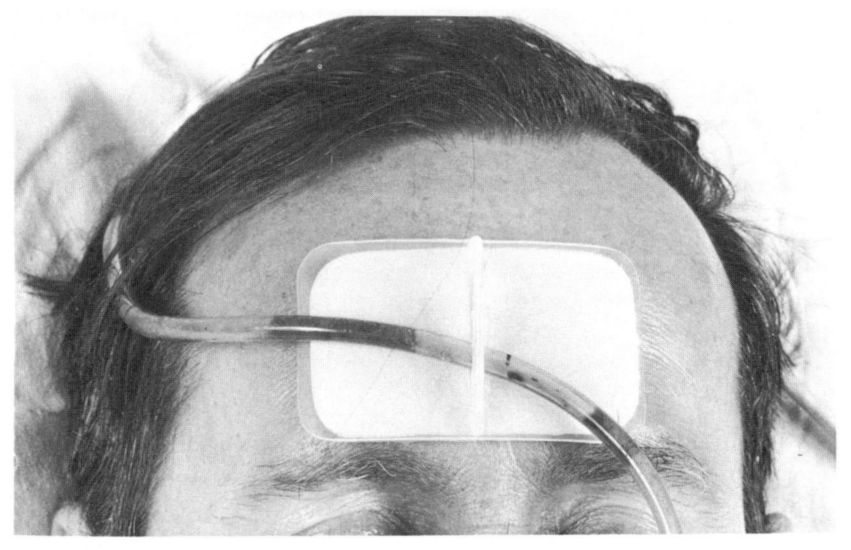

Fig. 10.1 A nasogastric tube held in position with a self-adhesive retainer.

Tube feeding is started gradually with water, followed later by milk and water or a dilute preparation of a diet, all at room temperature. During the initial period the tube must be aspirated hourly to ensure that the stomach is emptying. Feeding is increased progressively, up to full requirements, over a few days.

Once the full feed has been attained, it can be given either in the form of one- or two-hourly boluses or by slow continuous infusion. The latter is preferable because it reduces the incidence of diarrhoea. Feeding should be discontinued overnight to mimic a diurnal rhythm.

Type of tube feeds

Liquidized food

Simply blenderizing a hospital meal may be quite adequate, but it is impossible to know the exact amount of food supplied because inevitably some of it is left around the sides and blades of the blender. Generally, critically ill patients need a more accurate method of feeding than this because not only is the nutritional content important but also the water and electrolyte content.

Feeds based on milk

Many tube feeds are based on milk which can be prepared in different nutritional quantities and volumes, and in many instances is quite satisfactory. Table 10.4 shows the ingredients of a typical 3000 calorie diet, with 10 per cent of the calories obtained from protein, 50 per cent from carbohydrate and 40 per cent from fat.

Manufactured feeds

A number of nasogastric feeding preparations containing undigested ingredients are available, of which Complan and Clinifeed are suitable examples. If additional calories are required, they can be given as glucose by using Hycal, Caloreen or Calonutrin. Elemental diets

Table 10.4 A 3000-calorie milk-based tube feed

Preparation	Milk	Prosparol (fat)	Lactose (sugar)	Casilan (protein)	Water	Total value
Quantity	1000 ml	270 ml	250 g	35 g	1700 ml	3000 ml
Sodium (mmol)	22	–	–	–	–	22
Potassium (mmol)	41	–	–	–	–	41
Calcium (mmol)	8.16	–	–	–	–	8.16
Iron (mmol)	0.00105	–	–	–	–	0.00105
Carbohydrate (g)	48	–	250	–	–	298
Protein (g)	34	–	–	35	–	69
Fat (g)	37	135	–	–	–	172
Calories	660	1215	1000	140	–	3015

are also an effective nasogastric feed. Table 10.5 shows the composition of a 2600 calorie elemental diet.

Whichever type of nasogastric feed is used, it must not be too concentrated (hyperosmolar) but diluted with water to make the osmolality similar to that of plasma.

Table 10.5 Constituents of an elemental diet

Content			
Albumaid (protein)	Provides	Protein	60 g
Caloreen (glucose)		Fat	10 g
Triglyceride (fat)		Carbohydrate	560 g
Mineral mixture (major electrolytes)		Calories	2580
		Sodium	73.44 mmol
Ketovite (vitamins)		Potassium	21.29 mmol
Water (boiled) 2000 ml		Calcium	22.15 mmol
		Iron	0.30 mmol

Complications of nasogastric feeding

There are three main complications associated with nasogastric feeding.

1. Diarrhoea may become a problem with any type of feed. It is usually related to the high concentration (osmolality) of the feeds. If it develops, codeine phosphate linctus BPC, kaolin or diphenoxylate hydrochloride (Lomotil) may give control, but if these fail the diet will have to be diluted further or substituted by water for a period.

2. Oesophagitis can arise from pressure of the tube in the oesophagus and by regurgitation of acid from the stomach. It is a particular hazard in patients receiving steroids and can be a cause of severe bleeding. Alkalis and, more recently, the histamine antagonist, cimetidine, help in its prevention.

3. Inhalation pneumonia may be caused either by malposition of the tube or, especially in patients with an incompetent cardiac sphincter, by aspiration of gastric contents. In addition to confirming the position of the tube by standard methods, its radio-opaque tip can be seen on a chest x-ray and should be repeatedly checked.

Nasogastric feeding is a relatively inexpensive, simple and convenient way of providing nutritional support. It has adaptability, the ingredients may be altered to suit the individual needs and it can be used for prolonged periods in many cases. At times, however, it may not be possible to supply all the protein and calories required by nasogastric feeding alone. Tube feeding and an intravenous feeding regimen have then to be combined.

Although reference has been made only to nasogastric feeding, any of the feeds described can be used equally successfully via a gastrostomy or jejunostomy.

Intravenous feeding

This is always necessary for patients in whom it is physically impossible to pass a feeding tube, such as those with severe head injuries, or who are unable to absorb food from the bowel.

Intravenous feeding solutions

These consist of a calorie source, a nitrogen source with added electrolytes, vitamins and certain elements.

Protein solutions
Until very recently these consisted of two types, one a protein hydrolysate and the other a synthesis of individual amino acids. The hydrolysates have, however, now been withdrawn from the market. Some of the protein solutions have a carbohydrate, glucose or fructose added.

Protein solutions are contraindicated in patients in liver failure, because the damaged liver cannot utilize amino acids and hepatic coma may be precipitated or worsened. Caution is also necessary in patients with renal failure, for too much nitrogen will result in an increase of blood urea.

Carbohydrate solutions
Glucose is the most widely used source and is available in concentrations of 10, 20 and 50 per cent. The osmolality of the solution increases proportionately to the concentration of glucose; above 20 per cent, because of the hypertonicity, they are highly irritant to the lining of veins.

Glucose is dependent on insulin for its utilization, and because catabolic patients are relatively resistant to the action of insulin they require additional insulin, sometimes in large quantities, to metabolize the glucose. The soluble insulin can be added to the bottle or bag of glucose solution, given as bolus intravenous or subcutaneous injections, or infused continuously from a separate pump.

To determine the correct dose of insulin, blood glucose levels are measured and the urine is checked for glucose. Blood glucose levels are measured using a Dextrostix in conjunction with a reflectance meter; the urine is tested by the Clinitest method. At first the measurements are made hourly until the dose of insulin is established, after which four- to six-hourly estimations usually suffice.

Table 10.6 Intravenous feeding preparations (contents per litre)

Preparation	Type of solution	Calories	Nitrogen (g)	Glucose (g)	Sorbitol (g)	Ethanol (g)	Fat (g)	Glycerol (g)	Potassium (mmol)	Sodium (mmol)	Chloride (mmol)	Calcium (mmol)
Glucose 10%	Dextrose 10%	410	–	100	–	–	–	–	–	–	–	–
Glucose 50%	Dextrose 50%	2050	–	500	–	–	–	–	–	–	–	–
Synthamin 9	Sythetic amino acids	–	9.26	–	–	–	–	–	60.0	73	70	–
Vamin Glucose	Synthetic amino acids Glucose	650	9.40	100	–	–	–	–	20.0	50	55	2.5
Vamin N	Synthetic amino acids	250	9.40	–	–	–	–	–	20.0	50	55	2.5
Synthamin 14	Synthetic amino acids	–	14.30	–	–	–	–	–	60.0	73	70	–
Aminoplex	Synthetic amino acids Sorbitol 10% Ethanol 5%	1000	5.00	–	125	50	–	–	15.0	35	62	–
Aminoplex 14	Synthetic amino acids	340	13.40	–	–	–	–	12	30.0	35	81	–
Intralipid 10%	Soya bean oil Fractionated egg Lecithin 12 g	1100	–	–	–	–	100	25	–	–	–	–
Intralipid 20%	Soya bean oil Fractionated egg Lecithin 12 g	2000	–	–	–	–	100	25	–	–	–	–

Fructose is supplied in a 10, 20 or 30 per cent solution and is less irritant to the veins than is glucose.

Fructose is converted in the liver to glucose. This process is insulin independent; further metabolism is completely dependent on insulin because its utilization occurs as glucose. Therefore, these solutions seem to have no advantage over glucose and possess certain disadvantages such as the production of lactic acidosis, particularly in infants.

Sorbitol is a polymer of fructose and is prepared as a 30 per cent solution. It can only be utilized after its conversion in the liver to fructose; sorbitol is metabolized in the same manner as fructose and, therefore, suffers from the same disadvantages.

Alcohol solutions have the advantage of greater calorific value than other carbohydrate solutions and in some patients produce a euphoriant effect which may be beneficial.

Alcohol solutions should not be given to patients with liver or pancreatic disease but can be given to other patients with safety in amounts not exceeding 1.5 g/kg of body weight daily.

Fat solutions

These are prepared from two sources: soya bean oil (Intralipid) and cotton seed oil (Lipiphysan). In planning a feeding regimen, usually half the required calories are obtained from fat.

When a fat solution is given, it is important to check regularly that it is being utilized. This is easily done by inspecting a sample of serum—taken 12 hours after completion of the fat infusion—for milkiness or fat globules. If either are apparent, further fat solution is omitted from the feeding regimen. Fat is not included in the nutritional support of patients with significant liver disease because they are unable to metabolize it.

A large number of intravenous feeding solutions are commercially produced (Table 10.6). Examples of a moderate and high calorie feeding regimen are given in Tables 10.7 and 10.8.

Table 10.7 An intravenous feeding regimen

Solution	Volume (ml)	Calories	Nitrogen (g)	Sodium (mmol)	Potassium (mmol)
First infusion, over 12 hours					
Dextrose 50%	500	1025	–	–	–
Synthamin 9	500	–	4.63	36.5	30.0
Intralipid 10%	500	550	–	–	–
Second infusion, over 12 hours					
As for first infusion					
Total infused	3000	3150	9.26	73.0	60.0

Table 10.8 A high calories and nitrogen regimen

Solution	Volume (ml)	Calories	Nitrogen (g)	Sodium (mmol)	Potassium (mmol)
First infusion, over 12 hours					
Dextrose 50%	500	1025	–	–	–
Synthamin 14	500	–	7.15	36.5	30.0
Intralipid 20%	500	1000	–	–	–
Second infusion, over 12 hours					
As for first infusion					
Total infused	3000	4050	14.30	73.0	60.0

Method of administration

The dextrose feeding solutions have a high osmolality and are consequently very irritant, rapidly causing thrombophlebitis of peripheral veins. Therefore the solutions need to be given through a central venous catheter, and ideally the calorie and amino acid solutions are administered simultaneously to obtain maximum utilization of the feeding preparations. A four-way junction tube, Y-adaptor giving set or a ramp of stopcocks (Fig. 10.2) can each be used for giving solutions concurrently. The solutions are conveniently infused by an automatic drop counter, a continuous slow infusion pump or a burette-type giving set, all of which are ways of ensuring a correct rate of delivery. The hourly infusion volume is determined by dividing the volume of each solution by the number of hours in which it is to be given. The automatic drop counter is set to deliver the required number of drops per minute for the hourly volume and a burette or infusion pump is filled to the appropriate volume each hour.

The over-riding risk of intravenous feeding is systemic infection: the solutions used are ideal culture media for bacteria, the catheter provides direct access to the major veins and local infection around the catheter site can easily spread along the length of the catheter (Fig. 10.3).

At the first sign of inflammation around the infusion site or if the patient develops an unexplained fever, blood cultures should be taken and the catheter removed and its tip sent for culture.

The incidence of infection during intravenous feeding can be kept to a minimum but demands constant attention to the codes of aseptic practice.

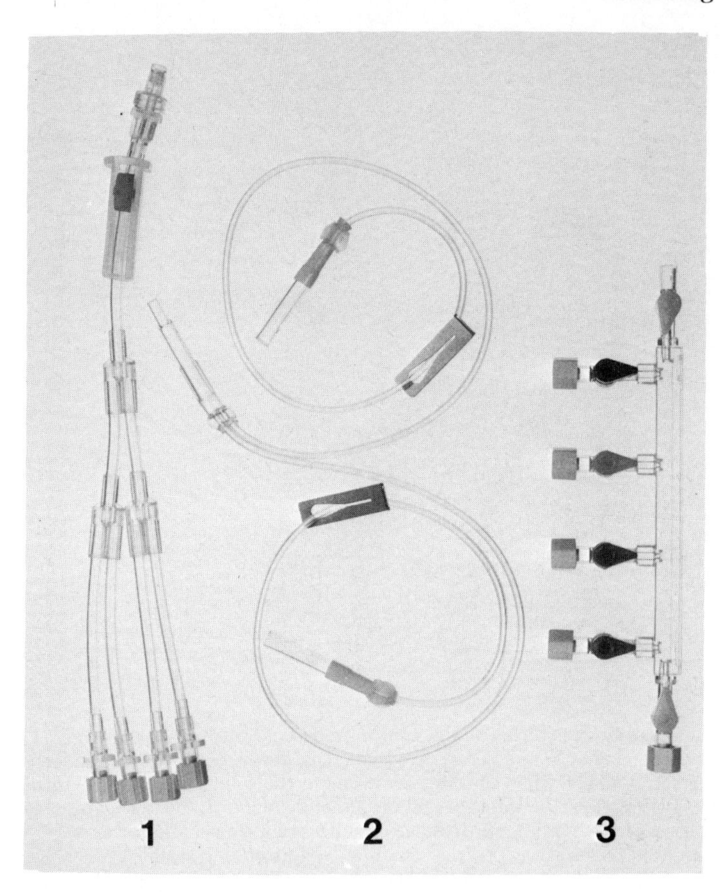

Fig. 10.2 Methods for the simultaneous administration of intravenous solutions: 1, four-way junction tube; 2, Y-adaptor giving set; 3, ramp of stopcocks.

Care of the catheter

The catheter may be inserted via the subclavian, internal jugular or antecubital veins. After insertion it is anchored in position by sutures and covered by a sterile dressing. If a transparent dressing such as Op-Site is applied, it need not be removed to observe the site of insertion for signs of infection, but only if it becomes non-adherent. Other types of dressings have to be renewed daily for this purpose. An antibiotic spray or ointment may be used to protect the infusion site before it is dressed but, in the absence of any firm evidence of their

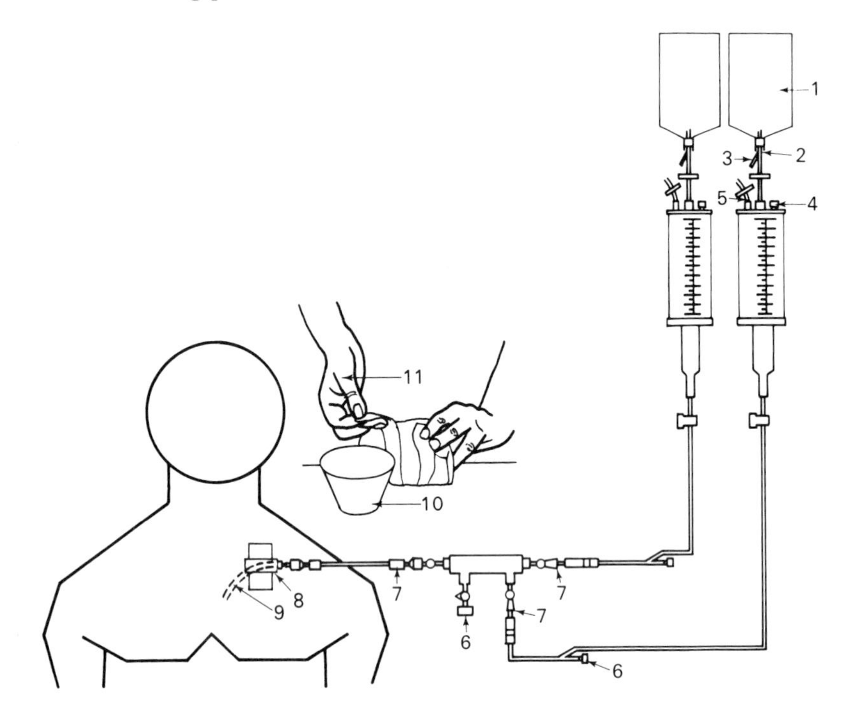

Fig. 10.3 Possible sites for bacterial contamination of intravenous therapy: 1, solution container: bottle cracked or polythene bag punctured; 2, during insertion of the giving set; 3 and 4, when making additions to the solution; 5, wet bacterial filter; 6, injection sites; 7, adaptors and other connections; 8, during manipulation and irrigation of the cannula; 9, leakage of fluid around the catheter site; 10, use of contaminated antiseptics; 11, from the hands of attending staff.

benefit, this is not considered to be a necessary routine practice. The dressing needs to be sufficiently occlusive to prevent contamination from other sources (for example, a tracheostomy which is in close relationship).

In addition to care of the catheter site, the following rules must be observed.

1. Use the catheter only for feeding.

2. Change the administration sets and connections daily and after a fat infusion.

3. Keep additions to the solutions to an absolute minimum, and add them aseptically at the time required.

4. Use a separate peripheral catheter for blood and plasma transfusion.

5. Do not withdraw blood samples from the line. Taking blood samples from central venous lines not only increases the risk of

infection but also leads to contamination of the specimens by the infusion fluid. It is a practice that should not be allowed.

The response of the patient to any feeding regime must be assessed. Weighing the patient, if practicable, is the easiest method. It is also judged from the results of biochemical tests, in particular the serum albumin.

11
Infection control

Infection control is extremely important in any hospital situation but assumes major significance in an ITU. Infection poses a constant threat to the critically ill patient and both its nature and methods of spread have to be understood.

Nature and spread of infection

Infection is produced by invasion of micro-organisms into any tissue. The resulting damage is associated with their multiplication in the tissues, to which a host response is mounted. The intensity of this response varies according to the immunological state of the particular host.

Infection can be acquired from either *endogenous* or *exogenous* sources.

In *endogenous infection* the organisms are transferred from one body site, where they may exist as commensals, to another where they act as pathogens. *Haemophilus influenzae* and pneumococci normally of low pathogenicity in the upper respiratory tract will invade and cause infection in the lower respiratory tract when the mucosal lining is damaged. Gram-negative infections due to *Pseudomonas aeruginosa, Klebsiella, Proteus* spp. and *Eschericha coli* are a major problem in ITUs. These organisms are normal residents of the gastrointestinal tract but may be transferred to other sites. For example, if the nurse does not wash her hands after giving rectal care, she may contaminate wounds, catheters or cannulae.

Exogenous infection occurs from sources outside the body—from other people, materials or equipment (cross-infection). Bacteria enter the body by inhalation, ingestion or inoculation. Cross-infection arises by direct or indirect contact or from airborne spread. Direct transmission of bacteria from the source to the host is most commonly via the hands of attending staff. Indirect transmission involves an intermediary such as a piece of equipment. Airborne spread is by the passage of droplets from one individual to another as in coughing and sneezing or dust inhalation.

In most instances the presence of infection cannot be diagnosed from a single criterion, either bacteriological or clinical; furthermore, it is important to differentiate between bacterial infection and bacterial colonization. Infection is diagnosed from a number of facts, such as fever and leucocytosis, in the presence of bacteria. Colonization is produced when the bacterial flora is altered and an overgrowth of a particular organism occurs with no clinical signs of infection. The dividing line between infection and colonization (Table 11.1) in critically ill patients is by no means simple. Such patients have reduced resistant mechanisms and may react atypically to infection.

Table 11.1 Indices of infection and of colonization

Infection	Colonization
Presence of white blood cells in specimen	No white blood cells in specimen
Heavy pure growth of bacteria	A light or mixed growth of bacteria
Changes in flora over a period of days	
Related symptoms of infection	No symptoms
Fever	
Leucocytosis	

Susceptibility to infection

For a number of reasons, seriously ill patients are susceptible to infection.

1. *Illness* of any cause is associated with a lowering of the natural resistance; the more severe the illness, the more marked is its effect.
2. *Invasive procedures* (Table 11.2) bypass the superficial barriers and facilitate the entry of bacteria into the body.
3. *Changes in the bacterial flora* arise from the use of antibiotics, especially those with a broad spectrum of activity. Sensitive organisms are suppressed and the growth of resistant types is encouraged.
4. *Drugs*—in particular steroids, cytotoxic drugs and immunosuppressive agents—interfere with the resistant mechanisms of the body.

Additional infection risks arise in emergencies such as cardiopulmonary resuscitation where it is not always possible to practice strict asepsis.

Table 11.2 Examples of procedures which break through the body's bacterial defences

Endotracheal intubation
Tracheostomy
Arterial cannulation
Central and peripheral vein cannulation
Urethral catheterization
Peritoneal dialysis

Control of infection

This is directed towards preventing the transfer of organisms from either endogenous or exogenous sources. Of importance in this respect are a well designed unit, a high standard of hygiene, proper observance of isolation techniques and bacteriological surveillance.

Design of the unit

The beds may be arranged in a single open area, individual rooms or a combination of both. A number of single-bedded rooms, at least one-third of the total, are essential for patient isolation. Sufficient space must be allowed around each bed area to accommodate the necessary equipment. Some of it can be conveniently mounted on a wall-rail system, behind the bed head. This makes cleaning easier, reduces dust accumulation and minimizes the need to move equipment. Each bed area must have its own hand-basin. Working surfaces and cupboards should be functionally designed so that they are easy to clean and maintain. Generous space should be allocated for dirty and clean utility rooms and for separate equipment storage rooms. To reduce the number of airborne organisms, a plenum (positive pressure) ventilation system which exchanges the room air 10–15 times every hour is advisable.

Hygiene

The incidence of infection is significantly reduced by careful attention to the practice of hygiene. This includes consideration of the environment, the staff and the patient.

The environment
It has already been emphasized that Gram-negative infections present a particular problem. These oganisms thrive in the many moist situations encountered in an ITU (Table 11.3). Many other objects

Table 11.3 Methods for combating bacterial contamination

Equipment/article	Frequency of changing	Methods of sterilization
Ventilator	Completion of use on a patient	1. Autoclavable respiratory circuit 2. Cycling formalin vapour through the machine 3. Cycling ethylene oxide through the machine
Ventilator respiratory circuit tubing	Daily	Autoclavable (tested afterwards for its anti-static properties)
Connections for endotracheal or tracheostomy tube	Daily	Autoclavable
Humidifier	Daily	Autoclavable
Heater for humidifier	Daily	1. Autoclavable 2. 2% Glutaraldehyde
Sterile distilled water for filling humidifier	Bottle discarded and replaced at least daily	
Respirometer	Completion of use on a patient	1. Cycling ethylene oxide through the respirometer 2. Cycling formalin vapour through the respirometer 3. Dry heat at a temperature not exceeding 70°C
Suction jars	Daily	Autoclavable
Suction tubing and connections	Daily	Disposable/autoclavable
Chest drain + tubing	Daily	Disposable/autoclavable
Oxygen masks	Daily	Disposable
Oxygen tubing	Daily	Disposable
Intravenous administration set	Daily, and after plasma, blood or fat infusions	Disposable
Three-way taps	Daily/more frequently if contaminated	Disposable
Drainage bag + tubing attached to collect excreta	Daily and whenever necessary	Disposable

(Table 11.4) are potential bacterial reservoirs. To prevent the dissemination of organisms from ventilators, bacterial filters can be attached to the expiratory port, or this can be connected to the outside.

Table 11.4 Reservoirs for bacterial growth, and methods for reducing it

Reservoir	Method
Hand-basins	Once in every 24 hours pour a 10% solution of sodium hypochlorite down the outlet and allow it to remain for at least 1 hour before flushing away
Tablet soap and its container	Instead use a 4% chlorhexidine gluconate solution detergent (Hibiscrub) or other antiseptic detergent
Patient's own toilet articles	Use autoclavable or disposable shaving kits and a disposable flannel and a solution of chlorhexidine plus cetrimide (Savlon) for washing the skin
Lubricating jellies Ointments Creams Antiseptics	Use single-dose applications but when this is not possible the appropriate application must be dispensed in a small container and kept solely for one patient's use
Water in flower vases	Discourage the presence of flowers in the unit
Free-standing water (e.g. water for flushing through suction catheters)	Discard after use

It is essential that a high standard of cleanliness of general surfaces, walls and floors is maintained. The daily routine for the domestic staff includes the cleaning of all surfaces with detergent and hot water, with particular attention to the ledges of doors, cupboards and windows. The floor must be vacuumed to remove dust and then washed with a detergent and hot water. Hand-basins and their outlets (ideally there should be no overflow) are cleaned with a powder or liquid containing bleach which kills the Gram-negative organisms lurking in these sites.

The nursing staff must be responsible for cleaning the equipment at each bed area. This is damp-dusted with a suitable disinfectant after the domestic staff have completed their duties. Phenolic compounds such as Hycolin 1 per cent or a 1 in 40 solution of Sudol are effective for this use. It is important that spillage of blood, bodily secretions, lotions or fluids is always removed immediately because each one is a source of contamination.

The unoccupied bed areas must be kept ready, so the daily cleaning routine is conducted in a similar manner.

Safe disposal methods for used items must be practised, with facilities at each bed area for disposing of all waste material. Separate, distinctive containers are necessary for used syringes, with puncture proof ones for sharp objects to avoid accidental injuries.

Staff
The hands of staff are the main vectors for transferring bacteria to either the patient or equipment. The need for frequent hand-washing with an antiseptic detergent, followed by thorough drying of the hands, cannot be over-stressed. It is the most important procedure in controlling contact infection. It must be carried out before starting and after completing every procedure to a patient and also when leaving one patient to go to another.

Symptom-free carriers of potentially pathogenic organisms are another hazard. *Streptococcus pyogenes* and *Staphylococcus aureus* are both risks because the rate of nasal carriage of these organisms is high amongst hospital staff. *Staphylococcus aureus* can also remain viable in dust on bed linen and clothing. To protect patients, no staff, irrespective of their grade, should be allowed to continue their duties while suffereing from diarrhoea, vomiting , infected skin lesions or upper respiratory tract infections.

Staff must be provided with a clean uniform each day, and for comfort the design of this often differs from the standard hospital uniform. Adequate numbers of uniforms must be supplied so that, when they become soiled during a shift, they can be changed.

All visiting staff and relatives entering the unit should remove their outer clothing and put on either a cotton or disposable gown or apron which reduces contact transfer of bacteria.

Patient
The skin needs to be kept clean and free from bodily secretions, and when either the bedding or a dressing becomes soiled it must be changed. Strict adherence to aseptic practice is necessary and 'clean' nursing procedures must always be done before 'dirty' ones to avoid bacterial transfer.

Isolation techniques

Infected patients require isolation to contain the infection (source isolation). Highly susceptible patients need to be protected against acquiring infection (protective isolation).

Source isolation
This is the segregation, into a room, of a patient who has a suspected or known infection. The precautions vary with the type of bacteria and its mode of spread. Table 11.5 lists the organisms that are frequently encountered in an ITU and the isolation techniques required to prevent cross-infection. The number of staff having contact with the patient should be restricted to those who are directly involved in the patient's care.

Whenever possible, disposable articles should be used for nursing infected patients. These include items of bed linen, gowns, instruments, trays and eating utensils. A separate set of domestic cleaning utensils is necessary for the room. When equipment cannot be completely assigned to one patient, or sterilized after use (for instance, the 12 lead ECG machine) it must be disinfected before being taken from the room. An appropriate method is to wipe the piece of equipment over with a 10 per cent solution of sodium hypochlorite and then wash it with hot water and detergent. The 'double bagging' technique is used for disposal of waste material for incineration, linen to the laundry and equipment for re-sterilization. For this method, plastic bags or sacks are kept inside the room; when full, they are securely tied and placed in a second bag or sack outside the room. This is then

Table 11.5 Guide to isolation

Micro-organism	Site of infection	Infected 'material'
Gram-negative bacilli (predominant *Pseudomonas aeruginosa* (occurs particularly in ventilated patients) *Klebsiella* spp. (associated especially with excessive antibiotic therapy e.g. ampicillin) *Proteus* spp. *Escherichia coli* 'Coliforms', including species such as Enterobacter and Citrobacter	Respiratory tract Urinary tract Intravenous catheters Surgical wounds	Moist secretions and discharges according to infected site
Bacteroides spp.	Deep-seated respiratory sepsis/Abdominal wounds	Self-infection no danger to others
Gram-positive coccus: *Staphylococcus aureus*	All sites and particularly pulmonary	Infected skin lesions, sputum, nasal and bronchial secretions
Beta-haemolytic streptococcus (BHS) BHS groups C and G	All sites	Sputum, nasal and bronchial secretions
Streptococcus pyogenes BHS group A	All sites	Sputum, nasal and bronchial secretions
Streptococcus faecalis	Urinary tract Endocardium	Pus from wounds
Streptococcus pneumoniae	Respiratory tract	Sputum, nasal and bronchial secretions
Streptococcus viridans	Endocardium	Blood stream
Gram-positive baccili: *Clostridia* spp.	Wounds	Wound exudate
Gram-negative coccus: *Neisseria meningitidis*	Meninges	Sputum, nasal and bronchial secretions
Tubercle bacilli *Mycobacterium tuberculosis*	All systems but primarily pulmonary, lymph nodes, bones and joints	According to infected site

fastened firmly and labelled. If linen is being transferred, the first sack is stitched with alginate thread which disintegrates in boiling water and avoids the laundry staff having to handle any infected linen. To distinguish between the various items that are sent from the unit, a coloured label system should be used.

Additional source isolation precautions are required when patients are admitted suffering from either infective hepatitis (hepatitis A) or serum hepatitis (hepatitis B). These patients are a danger to the staff caring for them. The hepatitis A virus is excreted in faeces and is usually spread to others via the faecal–oral route in food and water, but can be transferred parenterally. Hepatitis B virus is carried in the blood and is identified by the presence of hepatitis B antigen (HB_sAg or Australia antigen). The virus is transmitted via the blood

Mode of transmission	Isolation of patient	Gowns to be worn?	Masks to be worn?	Consider bacterial filter on ventilator?
All methods	Yes for *Pseudomonas* spp., *Klebsiella* spp. and any multiple resistant Gram-negative organism	Yes	Yes for respiratory tract infection during the performance of respiratory care	Yes for respiratory tract infection
Endogenous	No	No	No	No
Skin scales from infection lesions and droplets	Yes, if triply resistant or methicillin resistant	Yes, if isolated	Yes for respiratory tract infection during the performance of respiratory care	Yes for respiratory tract infection
Droplet	Yes	Yes	Yes for respiratory tract infection during the performance of respiratory care	Yes for respiratory tract infection
Primarily droplet but all methods possible	Yes	Yes	Yes for respiratory tract infections during the performance of respiratory care	Yes for respiratorv tract infection
Gut lesions or urinary tract to blood stream	No	No	No	No
Droplet	No	No	No	No
Via blood stream from mouth (teeth) or upper respiratory tract following surgery	No	No	No	No
From bowel flora or soil	No	No	No	No
Droplet	Yes until 24 hours after antibiotic therapy commenced	Yes, while isolated	Yes (filter type)	No
All methods	Yes for pulmonary or exudative lesions	Yes, if isolated	Yes (filter type)	Yes for pulmonary infection

stream but urine, saliva and other secretions are also possible sources. Patients who are asymptomatic carriers of Australia antigen also present a risk and certain groups have a higher carrier rate, viz:

1. jaundiced patients;
2. patients with liver disease;
3. drug addicts;
4. recipients of multiple blood transfusions;
5. patients treated by haemodialysis;
6. homosexuals;
7. people from developing countries.

On addmission, all such patients should be screened for Australia antigen and isolation precautions followed until the results of this are known.

Cases of hepatitis must be isolated in a single room and a notice, 'Hepatitis Risk', fixed to the door. Disposable long-sleeved gowns and gloves are worn for every procedure. Extreme care is needed with the disposal of needles (which must be discarded into a puncture-proof container), syringes, intravenous cannulae and intravenous administration sets; all are double-bagged and labelled 'Hepatitis Risk' before being sent for incineration. Every item, be it equipment for re-sterilization or waste material, should leave the room in this way. Any fabric or other absorbent material that becomes blood stained or soiled with excreta must be removed immediately and sent for incineration; therefore, when possible, disposable articles should be used. Spillage of blood or bodily secretions should be treated by adding sodium hypochlorite to the spilled fluid and cleared away with paper towels before it dries because of the danger of aerosol dissemination. Safe transport of specimens to the laboratories is essential; 'Hepatitis Risk' labels must be attached to the forms and specimen bottles, care being taken not to contaminate the outside of the bottles. Carriage to the laboratory is by the double-bagging technique, the form being placed in the outer bag.

Accidental inoculation of staff with Australia-antigen-positive blood via a needle prick or through cuts and abrasions is a real danger. If it occurs, the member of staff concerned must be seen by the occupational health department and considered for prophylactic administration of specific high-titre anti-HB_sAg immunoglobulin.

On completion of source isolation, the room is cleared and waste material, laundry and equipment for re-sterilization are sent from the unit using the double bagging technique. Disposable items, even if unused, should be discarded. The equipment that cannot be sterilized and the fixtures in the room are wiped over with a 10 per cent solution of sodium hypochlorite, rinsed and then washed with a detergent and hot water. Stainless steel apparatus must not be left soaking in sodium hypochlorite because it is liable to corrode. The walls and surfaces of the room are washed and the floor scrubbed with a 1 per cent solution of sodium hypochlorite.

Protective isolation

This is carried out to prevent patients with impaired immunity acquiring infection. The amount of protection required varies according to the level of risk involved.

A single room is always needed; hand-washing before entering the room and wearing gowns, gloves and masks by those attending the patient is sufficient for the patient on prolonged steroid therapy and neonates. Stricter measures are required for patients with marked alteration of the normal resistant mechanisms. Such situations arise in the severly burnt patient and those who are receiving immunosuppressive agents. It is necessary to sterilize or disinfect all articles coming into contact with the patient, which includes linen, amenities, food and drink. The number of staff attending the patient should be kept to a minimum and they must wear full protective clothing. This means covering the hair with a cap or scarf, wearing a filter mask and a sterile long-sleeved gown and gloves to avoid bringing contamination into the room from outside.

Isolator tents

These may be used for source or protective isolation, the advantage being that staff can remain outside the isolator, performing all necessary treatment through gloves welded into the sides of the unit (Fig. 11.1). They have been successfully used in the management of patients with burn injuries, those receiving cytotoxic therapy and following organ transplantation (protective isolation) and to contain highly infectious diseases such as Lassa fever (source isolation).

The nursing management of 'source' or 'protective' isolation must include constant reassurance and full explanation of the necessary precautions to the patient so that feelings and fears of leper-like isolation are dispelled.

Bacteriological surveillance

Certain specimens are collected for bacteriological culture. The reasons for this are twofold: first, to identify the causative organism in an infection and to determine its sensitivity to antibiotics and, secondly, to detect the early appearance of organisms in vulnerable sites. For the latter purpose, the specimens that are usually collected daily are samples of sputum and urine, swabs from tracheostomy incisions, discharging wounds and drain sites, and samples of dialysate fluid.

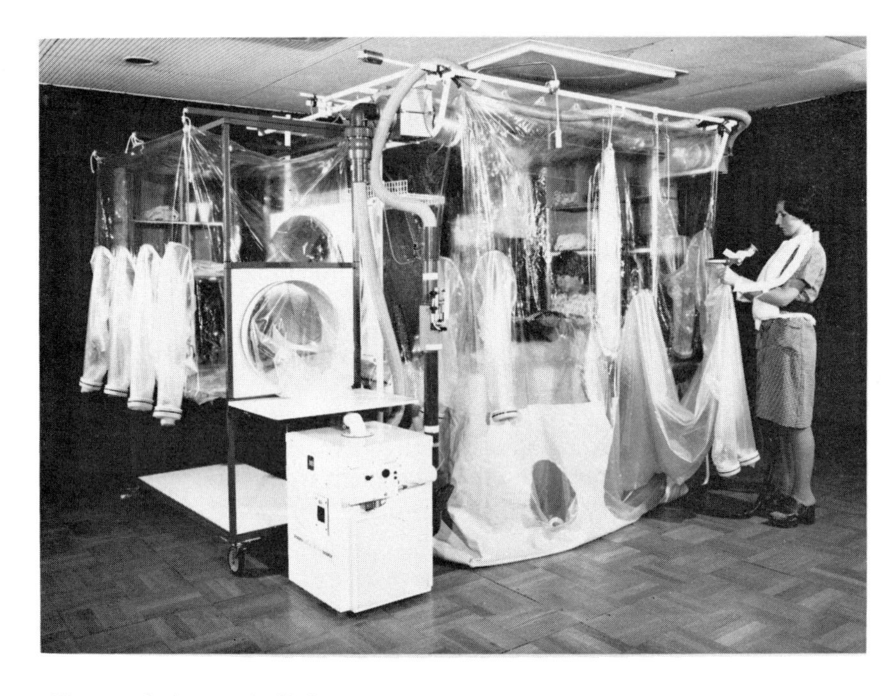

Fig. 11.1 Isolator unit (Vickers).

Section C
Cardiovascular failure

12

Dysrhythmias and conduction disturbances

The normal cardiac rhythm is sinus rhythm (that is, controlled by the SA node) with a regular rate of between 60 and 100 beats per minute. Dysrhythmias are disturbances of this normal rhythm and rate. They occur frequently in a wide variety of cardiac, respiratory and metabolic disorders. Their early recognition and treatment are of singular importance in the management of the critically ill.

Apart from the changes in heart rate associated with alterations in SA node activity, the dysrhythmias invariably arise from an irritable area of heart tissue discharging electrical impulses independently of the SA node. This constitutes an ectopic focus and can be situated in the atria, the AV node or the ventricles. Sometimes more than one may be present.

The site of the ectopic focus and the pattern of its electrical discharge determine the nature of the dysrhythmia. The reasons for their appearance are many but, in general, they arise either as a consequence of direct damage to the heart or because of changes in its chemical environment (Table 12.1).

Table 12.1 Causes of ectopic foci

Heart damage	Acute myocardial infarction Post-cardiac surgery Myocarditis
Acid–base and blood gas change	Acidosis Alkalosis Hypoxia Hypercapnia
Electrolyte changes	Hypokalaemia Hyperkalaemia
Drugs	Digoxin Isoprenaline Tricyclic antidepressants

Consequences of dysrhythmias

Some dysrhythmias have little impact on circulatory function whilst others cause a castrophic haemodynamic disturbance. The deleterious effects stem from:

1. Changes in the heart rate; the cardiac output falls at extremes of heart rate, both high and low.
2. Increased myocardial oxygen requirements and decreased coronary blood flow; because the heart rate is a major determinant of myocardial oxygen consumption and because coronary blood flow occurs mainly in diastole, both are adversely affected by rapid heart rates.
3. The loss of atrial transport function; the atria normally function as booster pumps. In diseased hearts the loss of this function can be significant.
4. The loss of synchronicity of ventricular contraction which interferes with their efficiency.

Classification of the dysrhythmias

The dysrhythmias are described in two groups, supraventricular and ventricular, according to their site of origin (Table 12.2). The supraventricular group is further subdivided into atrial and nodal (arising from the AV node).

Changes in the sinus rate, sinus tachycardia and bradycardia, whilst not strictly dysrhythmias, are included with the atrial group and classified as variations of impulse formation from the SA node.

Table 12.2 Classification of cardiac dysrhythmias

Supraventricular		Ventricular
Atrial:	Sinus tachycardia	Ectopic beats
	Sinus bradycardia	Tachycardia
	Ectopic beats	Fibrillation
	Tachycardia	
	Flutter	
	Fibrillation	
Nodal:	Ectopic beats	
	Tachycardia	
	Bradycardia	

Analysis of the ECG for dysrhythmias

This must be carried out systematically in line with the subdivisions of the ECG described in Chapter 2.

1. Look at a long length of ECG recording or a 'frozen' monitor display. Note if the rhythm is regular or irregular. If irregular, is there a repeating pattern (for example, coupled beats) or is it totally irregular, as in atrial fibrillation.

2. Calculate the heart rate by measuring the interbeat (R–R) interval, that is the distance between the peak of one R wave and the next. Convert this measurement to time (5 small squares (mm) = 0.2 second) and then to rate; for instance if the interbeat interval is 12.5 mm, it equals 0.5 second, and the heart rate is 120 per minute. If the rhythm is irregular, then the average duration of a number of intervals will give an average heart rate.

3. Note whether all the ventricular (QRST) complexes are alike. In supraventricular dysrhythmias, activation of the ventricles follows the normal pathways and the QRST complex is similar to that of a normal sinus beat. With a ventricular ectopic focus, activation follows abnormal pathways and produces different, sometimes bizarre-looking, ventricular complexes. This simple and usually obvious difference enables the dysrhythmia to be categorized into one of the two main groups.

4. Note the presence or absence of P waves. If present, observe their shape and their relationship to each QRS complex. Measure the P–R interval.

Working through this sequence will make it possible to reach a correct diagnosis in the majority of cases.

Individual dysrhythmias and their treatment

General indications for treatment

The mere presence of a dysrhythmia is not an indication for treating it. Many are transient and cause no problems. Treatment must be considered when:

1. The dysrhythmia is causing a deterioration of cardiac function.
2. An established dysrhythmia, if allowed to persist, will result in a deterioration of cardiac function.
3. Although causing no disturbance itself, it is a recognized forerunner of more serious dysrhythmias.
4. It is causing the patient distressing symptoms.

Whilst drugs form the mainstay of treatment, any associated metabolic disturbance must always be corrected.

Supraventricular dysrhythmias
Atrial

Sinus tachycardia

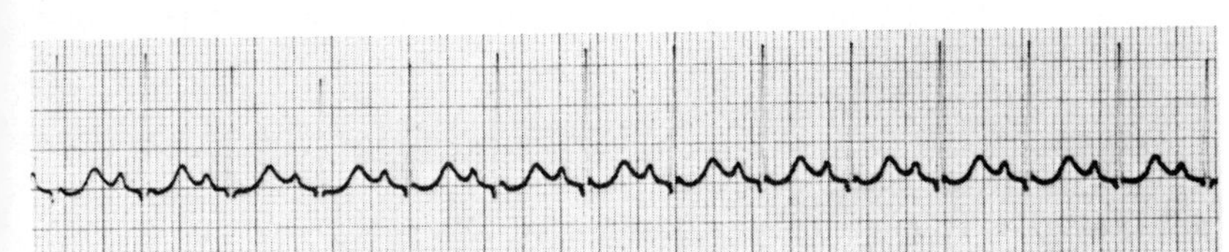

Fig. 12.1 Sinus tachycardia.

The SA node discharges at a rate greater than 100 per minute.

ECG diagnosis. Rate faster than 100 per minute (R–R interval $<$15 mm)
Regular rhythm
Normal QRS waveform
Normal P waves
Normal P–R interval

It is caused by a number of generalized disturbances such as anxiety, pain or fever, and develops reflexly in states of low cardiac output. Certain drugs (for example, isoprenaline and atropine) produce it, and it is a feature of hyperthyroidism. It has no haemodynamic consequences and treatment is that of the underlying condition.

Sinus bradycardia

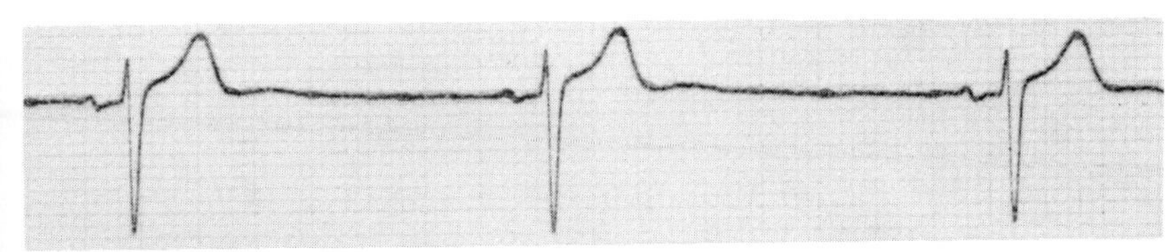

Fig. 12.2 Sinus bradycardia.

The SA node discharges at a rate of less than 60 per minute.

ECG diagnosis. Rate less than 60 per minute (R–R interval $>$ 25 mm)
Regular rhythm
Normal QRS waveform
Normal P waves
Normal P–R interval

Causes are:

1. An increase in vagal tone, provoked by fear, pain or, occasionally, tracheal suction.
2. Acute myocardia infarction; it is common in inferior myocardial infarcts because the artery supplying the SA node is often affected.
3. Drugs: morphine and the digitalis glycosides increase vagal activity; beta blocking agents.

Treatment. If there is no haemodynamic disturbance, nor associated ventricular ectopic beats, no treatment is required. However, sinus bradycardia can be associated with both of these complications, in which case atropine 0.6–1.8 mg intravenously will block the vagal tone and increase the heart rate. The effect of atropine is short lived and it may have to be given at frequent intervals. If it is not effective, then an infusion of isoprenaline or cardiac pacing may be needed.

Atrial ectopic dysrhythmias

In these, ventricular contraction is synchronous and the 'blocking action' of the AV node imposes an upper limit to the ventricular rate. These two factors help to offset their severity but they can still produce a rapid and marked circulatory disturbance.

Atrial ectopic beats

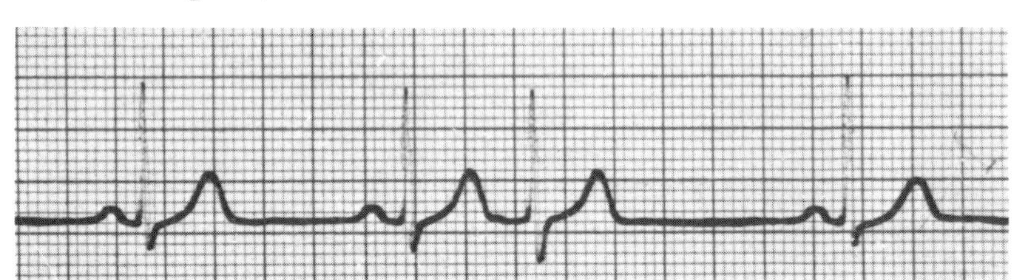

Fig. 12.3 Atrial ectopic beat.

These are common but rarely significant. They can occur in pairs and are one cause of a bigeminal rhythm; three or more consecutively constitute paroxysmal atrial tachycardia. An increase in their frequency may herald the onset of atrial fibrillation. No treatment is necessary unless the patient has unpleasant palpitations.

ECG diagnosis: Beats occur prematurely
May be followed by a compensatory pause
The P wave differs in shape from that of sinus origin
The P–R interval varies according to the location of the ectopic focus

Atrial tachycardia

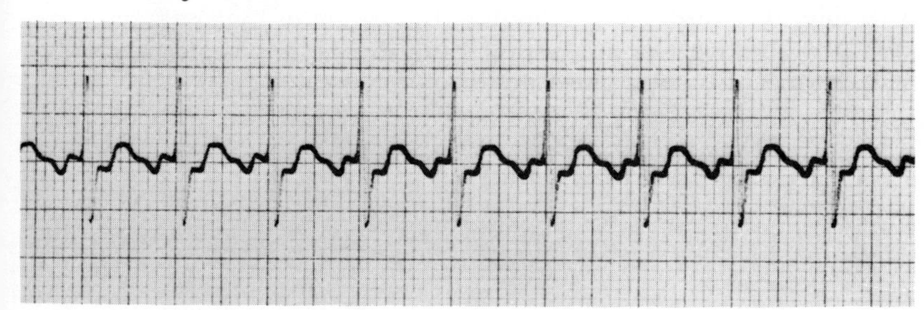

Fig. 12.4 Atrial tachycardia.

An atrial ectopic focus discharges at a rate between 140–220 per minute.

ECG diagnosis. Rate 140–220 per minute
Regular rhythm
Normal QRS configuration
The P waves are difficult to see because of the rapid rate. If visible, they precede each QRS complex

Differentiation from ventricular tachycardia. In ventricular tachycardia the ventricular complexes are abnormally shaped and are not preceded by P waves. The rhythm is also less regular.

Treatment. Short-lived episodes require no treatment. If the tachycardia persists it can cause unpleasant palpitations and may precipitate cardiac failure. Initially carotid sinus massage, with careful ECG monitoring, should be tried. If this fails then drugs that block atrioventricular conduction, and thus slow the ventricular rate, are used. Practolol (or other beta blocker) 5–10 mg, disopyramide 100 mg or verapamil 5–10 mg can be given intravenously. If long-term treatment is necessary, the patient is digitalized using digoxin.

Should drug treatment fail, a synchronized direct current (d.c.) shock can be given.

Paroxysmal atrial tachycardia with block

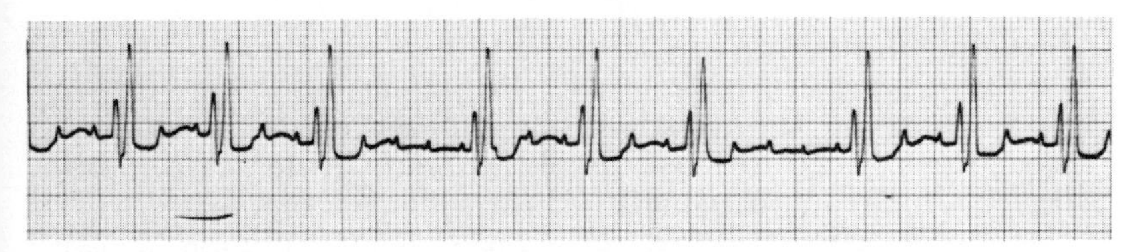

Fig. 12.5 Paroxysmal atrial tachycardia with block.

Because of impaired atrioventricular conduction, a number of the atrial impulses fail to reach the ventricles; the degree of block is variable. Its presence is a possible indication of hypokalaemia and digitalis intoxication. Potassium replacement may be necessary and withdrawal of digoxin is essential.

Atrial flutter

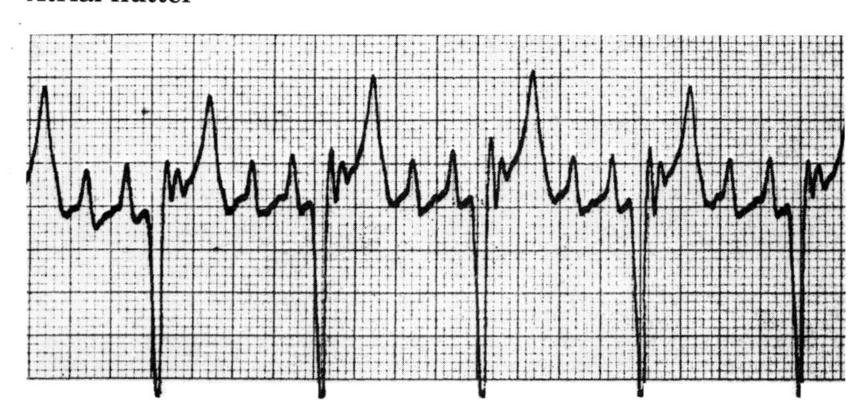

Fig. 12.6 Atrial flutter.

An atrial ectopic focus discharges at a rate between 250 and 350 per minute. Usually there is a degree of atrioventricular block, which can vary; 2:1 is common, giving a ventricular rate of 125–175 per minute.

ECG diagnosis. Rate depends on the degree of AV block
Regular rhythm
Normal QRS configuration
Flutter waves

The flutter waves are the cardinal feature. They appear as regular 'saw-tooth' undulations and the degree of atrioventricular block is expressed as the number of flutter waves to each QRS complex.

Treatment Atrial flutter usually requires prompt treatment. Drug treatment is the same as for atrial tachycardia; it responds readily to synchronized d.c. shock but carotid sinus massage has little effect.

Atrial fibrillation

This is a common acute dysrhythmia and, because of its association with chronic heart disease, many patients undergoing cardiac surgery are already in established atrial fibrillation.

An ectopic focus discharges at the rate of 400 per minute. At such a rate atrial function is disorganized and chaotic with no effective

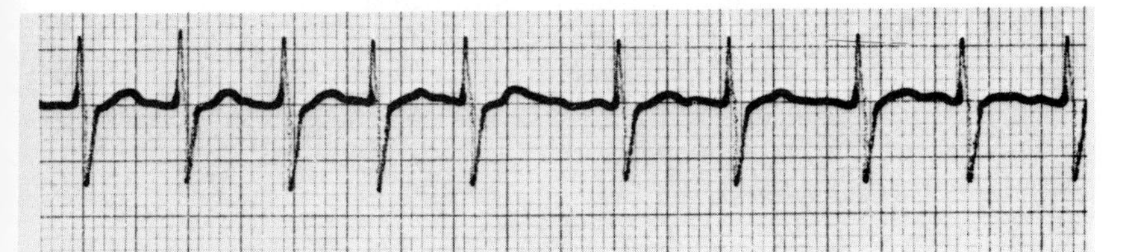

Fig. 12.7 Atrial fibrillation.

systolic contraction. It therefore predisposes to thrombus formation in the atria, with the associated risk of systemic and pulmonary emboli. The AV node is incapable of transmitting all the impulses and there is always a degree of block. This is variable and produces an irregular ventricular rhythm, usually at a rate between 120 and 150 per minute.

ECG diagnosis. Rate 120–150 per minute
Irregular rhythm
Normal QRS configuration
A fine fibrillary wave replaces the P waves

Treatment. If a rapid reduction of ventricular rate is required, any of the three previously mentioned drugs (practolol, disopyramide or verapamil) can be given. Digoxin is slower to act, but if the fibrillation persists the patient should be digitalized. The acute dysrhythmia may also respond to synchronized d.c. shock but its use in chronic atrial fibrillation has been largely abandoned.

Nodal ectopic dysrhythmias

Nodal ectopic beats

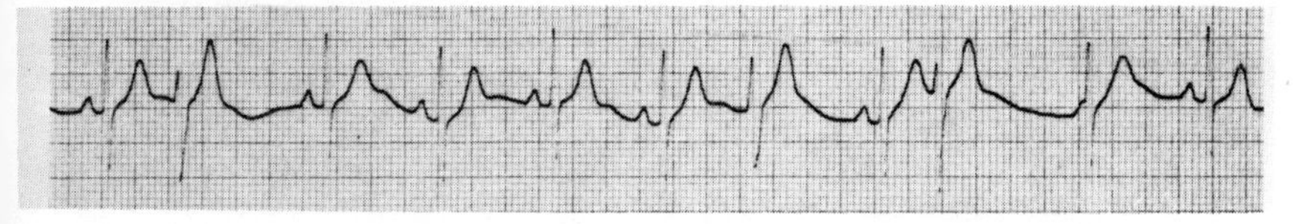

Fig. 12.8 Nodal ectopic beats.

These arise from a focus in the AV node and resemble those of atrial origin; three or more in succession constitute nodal tachycardia. Activation of the atria occurs in the opposite direction to normal and hence the P wave is inverted. The proximity of the ectopic focus to the ventricle results in a short P–R interval.

ECG diagnosis. Beats occur prematurely
May be followed by a compensatory pause

QRS configuration normal
P wave inverted
P–R interval short

The relationship of the P wave to the QRS complex is variable, depending on the position of the focus in the AV node. It may precede, follow or be obscured within it.

Nodal tachycardia

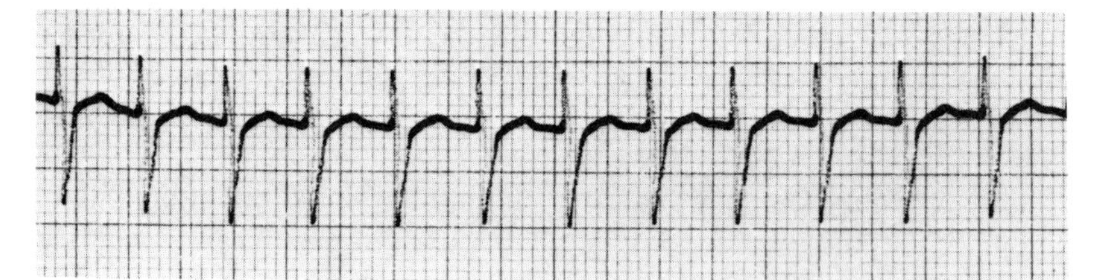

Fig. 12.9 Nodal tachycardia.

An ectopic focus in the AV node discharges at a rate of 140–220 per minute. It resembles atrial tachycardia and the treatment is the same.

ECG diagnosis. Heart rate 140–220 per minute
Regular rhythm
Normal QRS configuation
P waves not usually visible.

Nodal bradycardia (nodal rhythm)

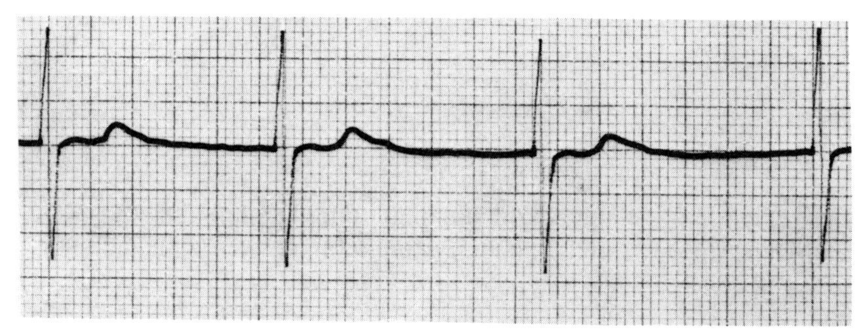

Fig. 12.10 Nodal bradycardia.

The AV node may itself become the pacemaker of the heart if the SA node is not functioning; during extreme sinus bradycardia it may 'take over' until the sinus rate increases. Digitalis toxicity is a common cause and treatment is with intravenous atropine.

Ventricular dysrhythmias

Ventricular ectopic beats

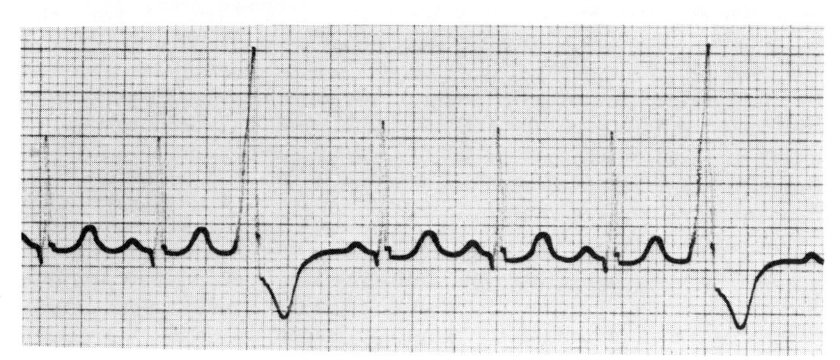

Fig. 12.11 Ventricular ectopic beat.

These are very common, especially after an acute myocardial infarction, following cardiac surgery and in association with hypokalaemia and hypoxia. In addition, a number of drugs, particularly isoprenaline, adrenaline and digoxin, may provoke them. As with all dysrhythmias, the frequency of detection depends on the efficiency of the monitoring.

Arising as they do from ectopic foci in the ventricles, the spread of electrical excitation is abnormal, the ventricular complexes are bizarre and muscle contraction is asynchronous. Ectopics from the same focus (unifocal) have the same ECG configuration but if they originate from more than one (multifocal) they will each differ in shape.

ECG diagnosis. Beats occur prematurely
Sometimes followed by a compensatory pause
Bizarre QRS complex with a wide QRS and a T wave pointing in the opposite direction.
No related P wave.

They may occur singly or in pairs and are the commonest cause of a bigeminal rhythm. Three or more in succession constitute ventricular tachycardia.

Ventricular ectopic beats, unless very frequent, cause no haemodynamic disturbance but their presence indicates ventricular irritability and the possible development of more serious ventricular dysrhythmias. There is an increased likelihood of this happening if they are multifocal in origin or occur in pairs.

R on T ventricular ectopics

During ventricular repolarization the heart is electrically unstable for a period corresponding in time to the crest of the T wave—the 'vulnerable period' of the cardiac cycle. A ventricular ectopic beat that coincides with this period (that is, an R on T ectopic) is likely to precipitate ventricular fibrillation. The relationship of ventricular ectopics to the T wave of the preceding sinus beat must be closely observed on the monitor.

Indications for the treatment of ventricular ectopics
Since they do not disturb circulatory function, ventricular ectopics do not require treatment; any treatment given is based on the premise that suppressing them will prevent or reduce the risk of ventricular tachycardia or fibrillation developing. Occasional unifocal ectopics are seen in 'normal' individuals.

The indications for instituting treatment relate to the degree of ventricular irritability:

1. If there are more than five ventricular ectopics per minute.
2. If they are occurring in pairs.
3. If they are multifocal, irrespective of the frequency.
4. If they are of the R on T type.

Treatment can be divided into three stages:

1. *Correction of general metabolic factors*, especially hypoxia, hypercapnia and hypokalaemia.

2. *Treatment of any coexisting bradycardia*. The association of sinus bradycardia and ventricular ectopics is common, particularly immediately after an acute myocardial infarction. Increasing the sinus rate with atropine will often eliminate the ectopics.

3. *Suppression of the ectopic focus*. A number of drugs can be used for this purpose. Lignocaine is currently the one of first choice: a bolus of 50–100 mg intravenously is followed by a continuous intravenous infusion at a rate between 1 and 4 mg per minute. Doses in excess of this may cause dizziness, paraesthesia and convulsions.

If lignocaine is ineffective then a number of other drugs can be tried, preference varying from unit to unit.

Mexiletine hydrochloride resembles lignocaine chemically but has the advantage that it can be given orally as well as intravenously. The dose by continuous intravenous infusion is 0.5–1.0 mg per minute.

Disopyramide is given intravenously in a dose of 100 mg followed by a continuous infusion at 20–30 mg per hour. It can also be given orally.

Procainamide can be given intravenously, intramuscularly or orally. Intravenous administration may cause hypotension and intraventricular conduction disturbances and it should always be given slowly. The dose is 100 mg per minute up to a total dose of 1 g. By continuous infusion the dose is 1–4 mg per minute.

Phenytoin is usually effective in dysrhythmias associated with digitalis intoxication. The intravenous dose is 50–100 mg repeated at 10-minute intervals until control has been achieved or a maximum dose of 1 g has been given.

Ventricular tachycardia

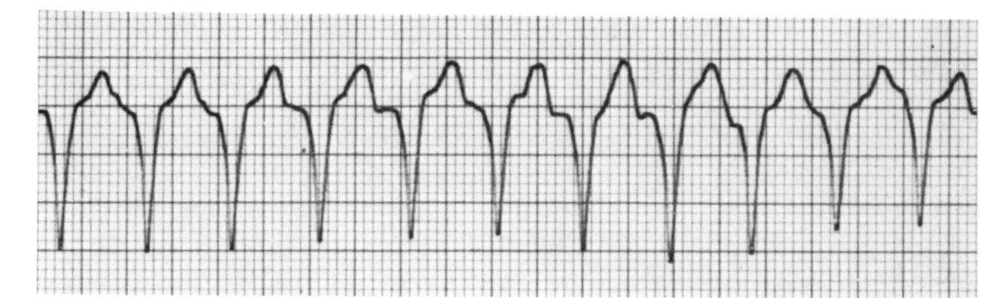

Fig. 12.12 Ventricular tachycardia.

Three or more consecutive ventricular ectopic beats constitute ventricular tachycardia, and its duration ranges from such very short episodes to attacks lasting several hours. It originates from a ventricular ectopic focus firing at a rate of between 140 and 220 per minute.

ECG diagnosis. The appearances are those of a succession of ventricular ectopic beats, broad bizarre QRS complexes and T waves pointing in the opposite direction. The R–R intervals are not absolutely regular and, although the atria continue to function independently under the control of the SA node, P waves are not visible.

Ventricular tachycardia is a very serious rhythm disturbance and, in combination with disease of the heart muscle, it causes a profound haemodynamic disturbance leading to cardiogenic shock or effective cardiac arrest. It may change to ventricular fibrillation at any time.

Treatment. This is always a matter of urgency. Lignocaine 100 mg intravenously should be given initially but if this fails, a d.c. shock should be given without delay. The subsequent treatment is as for ventricular ectopics, with continued suppression of the ectopic focus by a continuous infusion.

Ventricular fibrillation

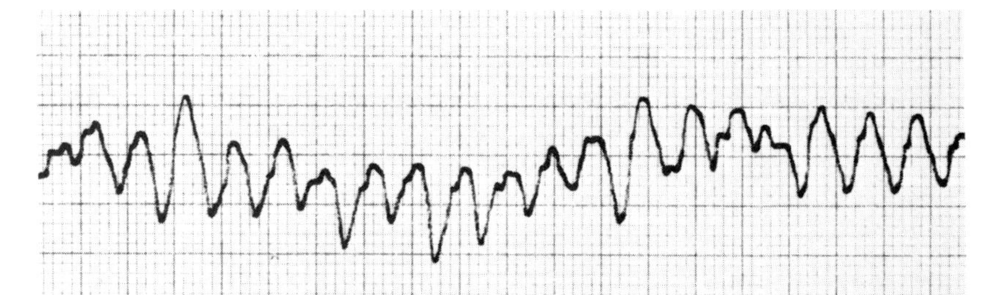

Fig. 12.13 Ventricular fibrillation.

This is one cause of cardiac arrest. The ectopic focus discharges at a rate of 300–500 per minute, and the ventricles can only respond to this in a rapid and chaotic fashion with no effective contraction.

ECG diagnosis. The trace shows an irregular series of deflections of varying height, width and shape. If larger, wider waves predominate, it is referred to as coarse ventricular fibrillation, in contrast to the fine type with small narrow waves. Its management is described in Chapter 13.

Atrioventricular (AV) block

This is characterized by a delay or interruption in conduction of the atrial impulses through the AV node and bundle of His. It is often referred to as heart block.

There are three grades or degrees of AV block.

First degree block

AV conduction is delayed but each atrial impulse results in a ventricular contraction. The ECG shows a prolonged P–R interval ($>$ 0.2 second) all P waves are followed by a QRS deflection (Fig. 12.14).

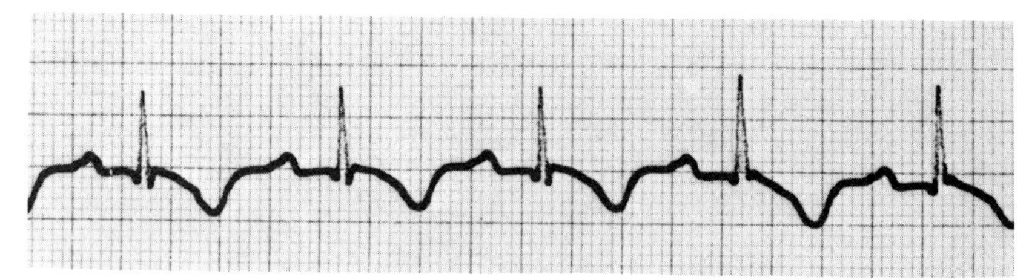

Fig. 12.14 First degree heart block.

Second degree block

There is intermittent failure of AV conduction when the atrial impulse does not elicit a ventricular response.

Not every P wave is followed by a QRS complex and the extent of the block is expressed as a conduction ratio. For instance, if there are two P waves to one QRS (that is, one impulse is not conducted) this is a 2:1 block; three P waves to each QRS (that is, two not conducted) is a 3:1 block (Fig. 12.15) and so on.

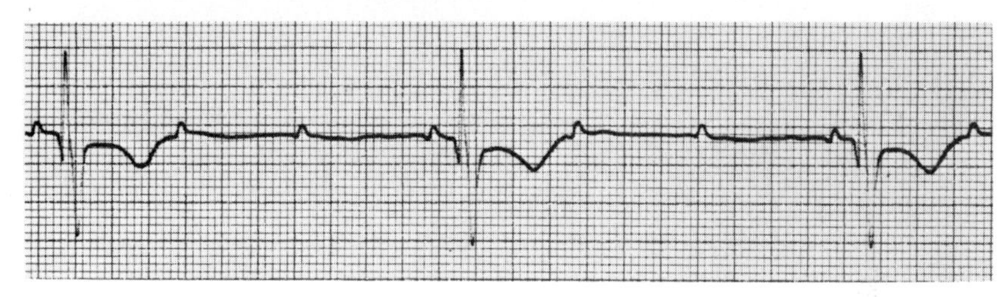

Fig. 12.15 Second degree (3:1) heart block.

One form of second degree block is characterized by a progressive increase in the P–R interval until an atrial complex is completely blocked—the Wenkebach phenomenon (Fig. 12.16).

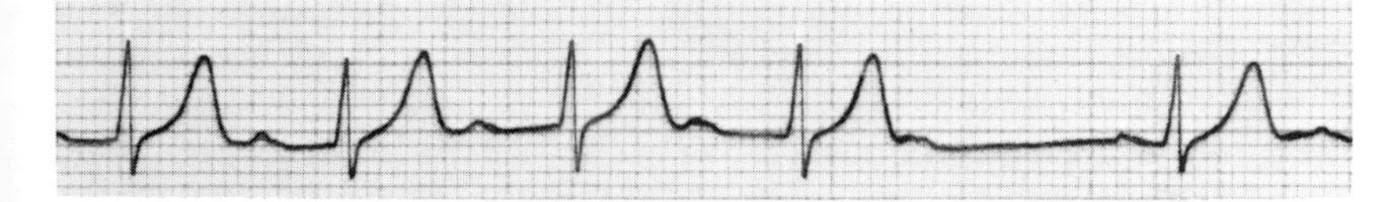

Fig. 12.16 The Wenckebach pnenomenon.

Third degree block

All supraventricular impulses are completely blocked and the ventricles beat independently of the atria. They are activated by a subsidiary ectopic pacemaker situated below the level of the block.

The ECG characteristics of third degree block (Fig. 12.17) are:

1. Complete AV dissociation; the P waves bear no relationship to the QRS complexes and reflect the higher atrial rate.
2. A slow ventricular rate, usually between 30 and 35 per minute; the more proximal the pacemaker, the higher the rate.
3. Abnormal QRS configuration; if the ectopic pacemaker is situated proximally, ventricular activation will be via the bundle of His, resulting in a near-normal looking QRS complex. If it is remote from

the normal conduction pathway, ventricular activation is abnormal and the QRS complexes are abnormal and wide.

First and second degree AV block are sometimes referred to as partial heart block, and third degree as complete heart block.

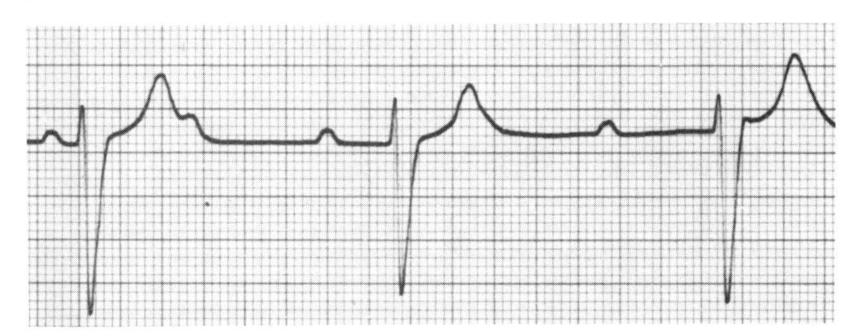

Fig. 12.17 Third degree (complete) heart block.

Aetiology

The degree of AV dissociation represents the severity of the conduction disturbance irrespective of its cause. A particular pathological lesion may cause any degree of block, which can vary if the disease progresses or improves.

The common causes are as follows.

1. *Acute myocardial infarction.* AV dissociation can occur with either acute anterior or inferior infarcts. When associated with an anterior infarct the prognosis is bad because of the likely large area of ventricular damage. By contrast, in inferior infarcts it is usually transiet and there is seldom a residual conduction defect.

2. *Following cardiac surgery*. Damage to the AV conduction tissue can occur during the repair of a ventricular septal defect or the removal of an extensively calcified aortic valve.

3. *Digitalis intoxication*.

4. *Inflammatory disorders* of the heart such as rheumatic fever and diphtheria.

Treatment

The presence of AV dissociation is not necessarily an indication for treatment unless the slow ventricular rate causes a low cardiac output or the ventricular rhythm is unstable (that is, there are periods of ventricular standstill, clinically apparent as Stokes–Adams attacks).

First degree block rarely requires treatment except to eliminate any direct cause, as in digitalis intoxication.

Second degree block, whilst not usually associated with circulatory disturbance, may progress to third degree block and some clinicians view this as an indication for inserting a cardiac pacemaker.

In acute third degree block, cardiac pacing is indicated, but if there are not symptoms and a high ventricular rate is present the pacemaker need not be activated.

In urgent situations before a pacemaker can be inserted, atropine, isoprenaline and adrenaline may all help to increase the ventricular rate.

Cardiac pacing

This section is concerned only with the use of pacemakers in the treatment of acute heart block.

The basis of a system for this form of cardiac pacing consists of a box that generates the pacing impulses and a catheter containing a wire with a terminal electrode to conduct these impulses to the heart muscle (Fig. 12.8). For reasons of electrical safety, external pacemakers are powered by batteries or rechargeable cells, not by the electrical mains.

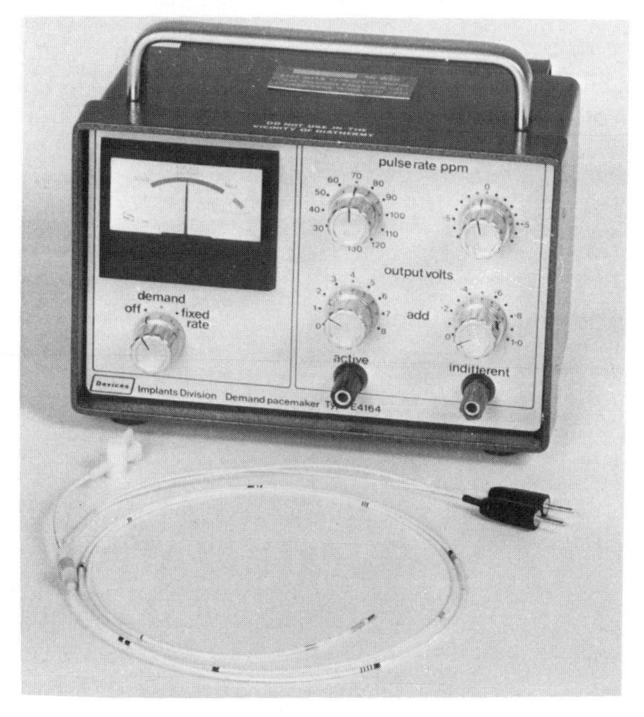

Fig. 12.18 A pacing box and catheter.

Endocardial electrodes are used, except in patients after cardiac surgery where wires are attached to the epicardium. The pacing catheter is inserted through a central or antecubital vein in exactly the same way as a catheter for measuring central venous pressure. It is advanced, with the help of x-ray screening, into the right ventricle where its tip is firmly positioned in the apex of the right ventricle. If x-ray facilities are not available, a flotation catheter with built-in electrodes can be used.

With the electrode in position, the catheter is attached to the pacing box. The controls for output voltage, rate and pacing mode are then set appropriately.

At the start the threshold voltage (that is, the lowest voltage that will pace the ventricles reliably) is measured and is usually less than one volt (1V); the actual pacing voltage is set at three or four times this value. The threshold voltage should be measured at least twice each day.

The choice of rate depends on the clinical situation; 70 per minute is usually adequate but higher rates (90–100 per minute) may benefit patients with heart failure. The pacing may be 'continuous' or 'on-demand'.

Sinus rhythm may return intermittently during recovery and there is then the danger of competition between the natural and the artificial pacemaker which might produce a very rapid heart rate or ventricular fibrillation if the pacemaker impulse falls during the vulnerable period of a normally conducted beat. Such problems led to the development of non-competitive, demand pacemakers. These incorporate a sensing electrode which detects the natural ventricular rate; if this exceeds the limit set on the box then pacing stops. A demand is therefore made on the pacemaker to operate below a certain natural ventricular rate.

Complications of endocardial pacing

There are three problems associated with endocardial pacing.

1. Displacement of the electrode causes a rise in the threshold voltage or loss of pacing.

2. Infection locally at the site of insertion is not serious, but spread along the catheter may cause a septicaemia.

3. Myocardial perforation; usually no harm results but the wire may need repositioning because of an unacceptable rise in pacing threshold.

Bundle branch block

This refers to a block of conduction in either the right or the left main branches of the bundle of His.

Right bundle branch block (RBBB)

Because the normal pathway for activating the right ventricle is blocked, it is stimulated from the left bundle via the septum; activation is therefore delayed and the QRS complex is widened and notched. Typically it has an rSR or M shape (Fig. 12.19).

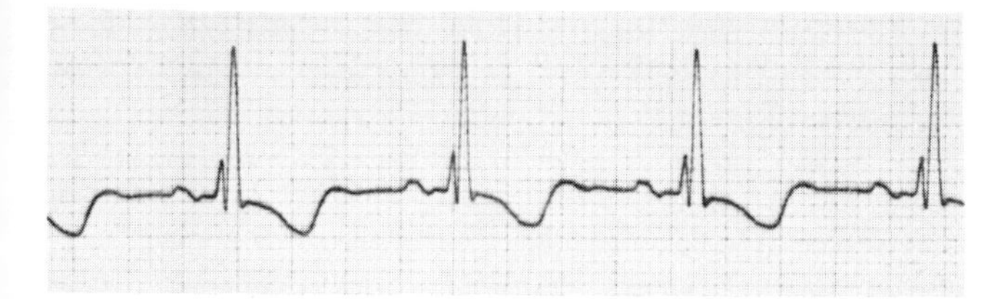

Fig. 12.19 Right bundle branch block.

Significance
RBBB is seen occasionally in normal individuals but its presence usually signifies some disturbance to right ventricular function. It may develop as a result of a myocardial infarction or pulmonary embolus, and is commonly associated with atrial septal defect and right ventricular hypertrophy of any cause.

Left bundle branch block (LBBB)

The left ventricle is activated from the right bundle by impulses passing to the left side of the septum below the block. Activation of the left ventricle is delayed, resulting in a widened, sometimes notched, QRS complex (Fig. 12.20).

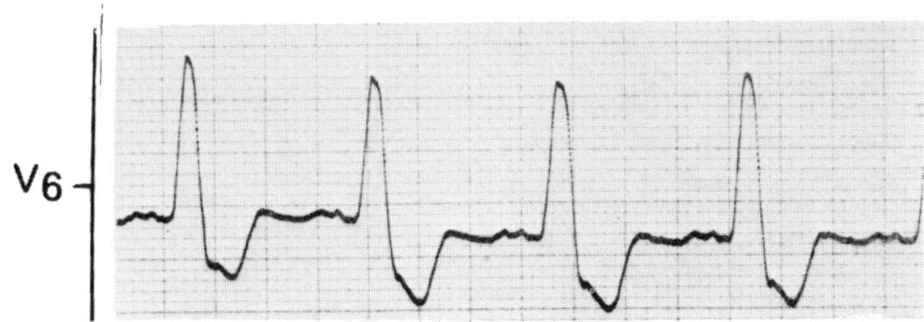

Fig. 12.20 Left bundle branch block.

Significance
LBBB always indicates organic heart disease. It is commonly associated with ischaemic and hypertensive heart disease.

Fascicular blocks

The left bundle has two discrete branches, anterior and posterior. Conduction can be blocked in either, leading to left posterior or anterior fascicular (hemi-) block. These can be recognized from the ECG.

A combination of RBBB and a left hemiblock means that only one conducting fascicle is functioning, and that there is a high risk of third degree AV block developing.

13
Cardiac arrest

The term 'cardiac arrest', although widely used, is partly a misnomer because only in complete asystole does the heart actually arrest. Its meaning, however, is widely understood as indicating an acute arrest of cardiac function with no effective circulation.

It can exist in association with:

1. Ventricular fibrillation.
2. Ventricular asystole.
3. Ventricular tachycardia.
4. Extreme bradycardia.

In the majority of instances ventricular fibrillation or asystole are responsible, although the relative frequency of each varies in reported series.

Aetiology

Cardiac arrest has many causes:

1. Acute myocardial infarction.
2. Hypoxia.
3. Hypercapnoea
4. Electrolyte and acid–base disturbances.
5. Pulmonary embolism.
6. Pericardial tamponade.
7. Drugs.
8. Hypothermia.
9. Electrocution.

Clearly a number of these may coexist in a critically ill patient and their effects will be cumulative.

Both hypo- and hyperkalaemia can cause arrest; the latter cause may be due to acute renal failure, rapid transfusion of bank blood or too rapid intravenous administration of potassium chloride.

A number of drugs, given or taken in excess, can also cause an arrest. They include digitalis, the toxicity of which is increased by hypokalaemia, isoprenaline which can cause ventricular fibrillation, and the tricyclic antidepressants.

In hypothermic patients, if the body temperature falls below 30°C the risks of ventricular fibrillation are greatly increased.

Clinical features

Loss of consciousness—unless, as may be the case in an ITU, the patient is already in coma, heavily sedated or paralysed on a ventilator.

Loss of major (femoral and carotid) arterial pulses. Respiration stops within 15–30 seconds after the cardiac arrest unless a respiratory arrest is the primary event. The pupils start to dilate after about a minute.

If the patient is being continuously observed and monitored, the arrest and its associated ECG changes should be recognized immediately. If the arterial pressure is also being monitored, the contour of the pressure waveform will be lost. It is most important to realize that the chance of successful resuscitation diminishes rapidly with the passage of time and any delay in restoring the circulation increases the risk of subsequent cerebral damage. ITUs must be highly organized to institute corrective measures immediately.

Management

The approach to resuscitation will depend on the setting in which the arrest occurs and also on its aetiology.

Immediate—if the arrest is due to ventricular fibrillation or tachycardia, two or three strong blows to the sternum may restore sinus rhythm and this manoeuvre should always be tried. If this is unsuccessful the emergency measures, described as the ABC of treatment, are started.

A clear the Airway
B institute Breathing
C establish a Circulation

Once the airway has been cleared, immediate ventilation can be achieved by inserting a plastic airway into the mouth and firmly applying over it a facemask connected to a self-inflating bag supplied with oxygen at a flow of 12–15 litres per minute.

Maintenance of an adequate circulation requires effective external cardiac massage given in the standard manner. Compression of the chest must be rhythmic, at a rate of approximately 60 per minute, with a constant relationship (5:1) to each inflation of the lungs. The sternum needs to be depressed between 3.5 and 5 cm.

Whilst external cardiac massage generally is a safe procedure, it should not be done too vigorously, especially in children. A number of complications can occur, including fractured ribs, haemothorax, pneumothorax, gastric rupture and laceration of the liver and spleen.

If an intravenous infusion is not already in place, one should be established, initially using 5 per cent dextrose. In collapsed patients, cannulation of a peripheral vein may not be possible and a central one has to be used. An arterial blood sample is required as soon as possible to measure the blood gas tensions, the acid-base state and the serum potassium. Numerous samples are often needed during the course of a resuscitation and the insertion of an arterial line can obviate the need for repeated arterial punctures.

Once these measures have been achieved, further management may entail:

1. Specific treatment of the underlying rhythm disturbance.
2. Endotracheal intubation and ventilation.
3. Correction of metabolic disturbances.
4. Treatment of cerebral oedema.

Treatment of the underlying rhythm disturbance

Ventricular fibrillation

A bolus dose of lignocaine (1.5 mg/kg body weight) can be given immediately; this may suppress the fibrillation and restore sinus rhythm. The essential treatment is *defibrillation*, using a direct current (d.c.) defibrillator (Fig. 13.1) set at 200 joules (J) for the first

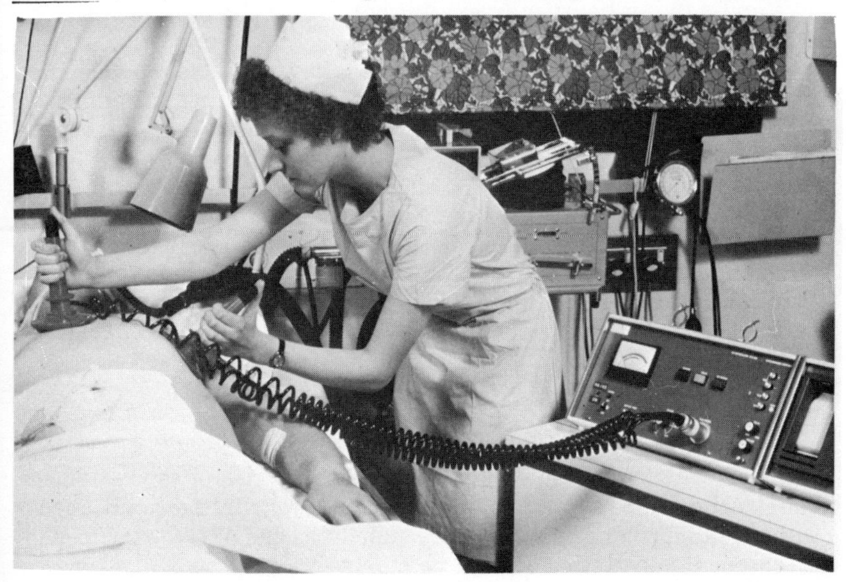

Fig. 13.1 Defibrillation.

shock in an adult. The paddles must be well coated with a conductive gel to ensure effective contact with the skin; the gel must not flow across the skin from one paddle to the other for this will form a low resistance pathway for the current, reduce the efficacy of the shock and might result in burning of the skin. One defibrillator paddle is positioned over the apex of the heart and the other to the right of the upper part of the sternum. All personnel involved should be warned when the shock is to be given so that they may stand away from the bed. If the first shock is unsuccessful, the shock strength is doubled to 400 J and repeated. Should fibrillation persist, its character must be noted; if of a fine pattern, it should be coarsened, using intravenous adrenaline, isoprenaline or calcium chloride, before the next shock is given. Correction of any abnormal metabolic factors is most important in the management of resistant or recurrent ventricular fibrillation.

Ventricular tachycardia
Lignocaine and d.c. shock are used as for ventricular fibrillation. Conversion to sinus rhythm usually occurs much more readily.

Asystole
This also includes extreme bradycardia which causes the clinical picture of cardiac arrest. Successful resuscitation from an asystolic arrest is less frequent than from one due to ventricular fibrillation, as it is usually associated with more extensive cardiac damage. Ventricular fibrillation and asystole are not, however, mutually exclusive and a dying heart may exhibit both, with the asystolic periods becoming progressively longer.

To treat asystole, some or all of the following intravenous drugs may be needed, often in repeated doses: atropine 2 mg, adrenaline 5 ml of 1 in 1000 solution, isoprenaline 2.5 mg and calcium gluconate 10 ml of a 10 per cent solution.

Ideally, they should all be given directly into the heart through a central venous catheter. The use of a long needle inserted through the chest wall into the left ventricle is less satisfactory because of the risk of damage to the myocardium and coronary arteries.

If these drugs are not effective, cardiac pacing can be tried but is rarely of any value.

Endotracheal intubation and ventilation

If the airway is inadequate or is threatened by risk of aspriation, an endotracheal tube should be inserted. Hand ventilation can be maintained but if prolonged respiratory support seems likely to be needed, mechanical ventilation should be started.

Patients who have frequent, recurrent episodes of cardiac arrest are better maintained on a ventilator; this allows the patient to be heavily sedated, and minimizes the great fear and anxiety they would otherwise experience.

Correction of metabolic disturbances

Acidosis

The acidosis is a consequence of the circulatory arrest. Lactic acid accumulates in the blood, causing a metabolic acidosis. If ventilation is inadequate there will also be some degree of respiratory acidosis due to the elevated P_{CO_2}.

Intravenous sodium bicarbonate in an 8.4 per cent solution is used to correct the metabolic acidosis. An initial dose of 50 mmol is given, followed if necessary by further amounts according to the measured acid–base state of the blood. During resuscitation there is a frequent and dangerous tendency to give too much sodium bicarbonate. This must be avoided because its high content of sodium (1000 mmol/litre) can overload an already damaged heart, producing pulmonary oedema or give rise to a hyperosmolar state. The high osmolality (2008 mmol/kg) of the 8.4 per cent solution also means that it is extremely irritant and inadvertent administration into the subcutaneous tissues can lead to unpleasant 'chemical burns'.

If the P_{CO_2} is high, it can be lowered by increasing the pulmonary ventilation.

Potassium

Hypokalaemia requires intravenous potassium chloride, usually at a rate of 10–20 mmol per hour.

Hyperkalaemia can usually be temporarily corrected with glucose and insulin.

Treatment of cerebral oedema

A period of cerebral hypoxia causes cerebral oedema, which should be treated with dexamethasone 10 mg intravenously. If the oedema is judged to be severe then this is continued, 4 mg six-hourly for 48 hours.

Open cardiac resuscitation

Closed-chest cardiac massage, if carried out properly, is most effective and can sustain an adequate circualation for long periods. It has replaced internal cardiac massage except in the specific instances where cardiac arrest occurs in postoperative cardiac surgical patients, associated with either cardiac tamponade or major haemorrhage. The complications are usually recognized before an arrest occurs and the patient can be transferred back to the operating theatre. On occasions, however, it will be necessary to re-open the chest in the ITU.

Abandoning resuscitation

This can be a most difficult and taxing decision to make, even for someone with great experience in managing cardiac arrest. There are no specific guidelines as to how long efforts should be continued to restore an effective heart beat, but the longer it resists treatment the less likely is a successful outcome. The cause of the arrest, the age of the patient, the presence of disease in other systems and evidence of neurological damage will all influence judgement.

Determining the severity of irreversible neurological damage can also be difficult at the time of resuscitation. Severe damage is suggested by deep coma, lack of spontaneous movement, lack of spontaneous respiration and fixed dilated pupils. None of these, however, at this stage, is an absolute sign and, if an adequate circulation has been restored, neurological assessment should be made later after cerebral oedema has been treated.

14

Shock

The meaning of the term 'shock' is controversial and knowledge of its pathophysiology is still incomplete. It is best considered as a syndrome in which there is an inadequate blood supply to the tissues to a level which is incompatible with normal tissue oxygen consumption, and where functional and structural changes occur in certain essential organs. It is therefore a disorder of blood *flow*, not blood *pressure*, and its diagnosis must be based on clear clinical and laboratory evidence of reduced tissue perfusion. It affects all the major systems and its management highlights the practice of intensive therapy.

Aetiology

A simple classification of the causes of shock is given in Table 14.1. Whilst three separate categories are described, there are, in practice, many instances where they overlap.

Table 14.1 Classification of shock

Hypovolaemic	Blood loss Plasma loss Extracellular fluid loss
Cardiogenic	'Pump failure' Dysrhythmias Pericardial tamponade Pulmonary embolism
Bacteraemic	Gram-negative infection Gram-positive infection

Hypovolaemic shock

This is caused by a reduction in the circulating blood volume, which can arise from loss of whole blood, plasma or extracellular fluid.

Gastrointestinal haemorrhage and multiple injuries are familiar examples of whole blood loss; severe burns result in a large loss of plasma, and depletion of extracellular fluid occurs when excess salt and water are lost as in severe vomiting or diarrhoea. When the clinical signs of shock first appear, a large reduction (up to 20 per cent) of the blood volume has already occurred.

Cardiogenic shock

Stemming from a reduction in cardiac output, cardiogenic shock most commonly develops after a severe myocardial infarction where the extensive damage of the left ventricular muscle compromises the pumping action of the heart. When the picture appears, around 25 per cent of the left ventricular myocardium has been affected. It also occurs after open-heart surgery and is a constant feature of pericardial tamponade and massive pulmonary embolism. The occurrence of cardiac dysrhythmias in any of these conditions accentuates the circulatory disturbance.

Bacteraemic shock

This is caused by bacterial toxins liberated from organism multiplying in the circulation.

Nowadays these are mainly Gram-negative bacteria, but Gram-positive bacteria can be responsible (Table 14.2). Gram-negative bacteria liberate their toxin when they die and it is therefore termed an endotoxin; Gram-positive bacteria actively secrete an exotoxin.

Table 14.2 Organisms that may cause bacteraemic shock

Gram-positive	Gram-negative
Staphylococcus aureus	*Escherichia coli*
Streptococcus pneumoniae	*Pseudomonas*
	Klebsiella
	Serratia
	Proteus
	Enterobacter
	Bacteroides

The features of bacteraemic shock are attributable to the action of these toxins on the cardiovascular and respiratory systems. They cause widespread vasoconstriction, increased capillary permeability with loss of plasma from the circulation and myocardial depression. It may occur as a complication of renal, abdominal, pelvic or wound infection, often after some form of surgical intervention and is a constant threat in patients with severe burns (Table 14.3). Whilst it is more frequent in surgical patients, 'medical' patients are not immune and those with diabetes mellitus, hepatic cirrhosis or impaired immunity are particularly at risk.

Table 14.3 Clinical associations and predisposing factors

Site of origin	Clinical association	Predisposing factors	Organism
Biliary tract	Cholangitis	Stones Surgery	*Escherichia coli* *Klebsiella* *Bacteroides* *Pseudomonas*
Bowel	Infarction Obstruction Perforation		
Urinary tract	Pyelitis Prostatic obstruction	Indwelling catheters Instrumentation	*Escherichia coli* *Proteus* *Klebsiella* *Pseudomonas*
Reproductive system	Surgery Abortion Postpartum		*Escherichia coli* *Bacteroides* *Clostridia* *Streptococcus*
Respiratory tract	Severe pneumonia	Endotracheal tubes Tracheostomy Ventilatory equipment Use of antibiotics	*Escherichia coli* *Klebsiella* *Pseudomonas* *Enterobacter* *Pneumococcus* *Staphylococcus*
Vascular system	Surgery/prosthesis Drug addiction	Central venous catheters	*Staphylococcus* *Escherichia coli* *Serratia*
Skin	Burns		*Pseudomonas*

The prognosis in bacteraemic shock depends more on the origin of the infection, the underlying clinical process and the patient's defence mechanisms than on the severity of the acute haemodynamic disturbance. It remains a very serious condition, and the mortality in various reported series of cases varies from 30 per cent to 80 per cent.

Pathogenesis

Similar mechanisms underlie the circulatory disturbance in all forms of shock (Fig. 14.1). The end-result is always a reduction in cardiac output due either to a decrease in the venous return to the heart or to damage to the heart muscle. The low cardiac output provokes an increase in sympathetic nervous activity and a release of catecholamines from the adrenal glands. The effect of these is to increase heart rate and myocardial contractility and to constrict the arterioles, particularly those of the cutaneous, splanchnic and renal circulations. The reduced peripheral blood flow decreases oxygen supply to the tissues; cell metabolism is affected and lactic acid accumulates, producing a metabolic acidosis. The combined affects of hypoxia and acidosis further slow the capillary circulation and increase the permeability of the capillary walls, with loss of plasma into the interstitial spaces. As a result, venous return and cardiac output are progressively reduced and a vicious circle is established which, if not interrupted, will lead to the patient's death.

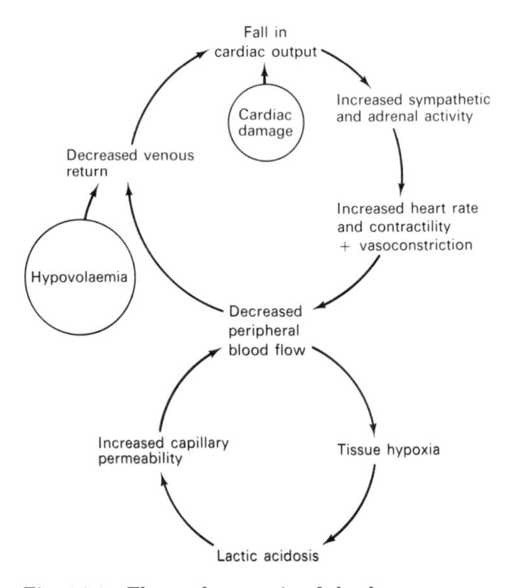

Fig. 14.1 The pathogenesis of shock.

Clinical features

These reflect the low cardiac output and increased sympathoadrenal activity. The patient is restless, sometimes confused or somnolent, pale and sweating with cold extremities and peripheral cyanosis. The pulse is rapid and of low volume, and irregularities signify the presence of dysrhythmias; blood pressure is usually low but can be normal if the increased peripheral resistance compensates for the low cardiac output. The urine output is reduced.

In cardiogenic shock there may be signs of pulmonary oedema and an elevated jugular venous pressure.

In the early stages of bacteraemic shock the picture may be somewhat different. The patient is hypotensive but has a warm pink skin (hot shock) and does not look particularly ill. It appears because circulating endotoxin sometimes has an initial vasodilator effect; the more characteristic features soon supervene.

General management

Frequent and detailed observations of the function of the vital systems forms the basis for good management. Clinical assessment alone is inadequate and has to be supplemented by:

1. Continuous ECG monitoring.
2. Measurement of central venous and/or pulmonary wedge pressure.
3. Frequent manual recording of arterial blood pressure or continuous measurement via an arterial cannula. Cuff pressure measurements are difficult to make and are unreliable in hypotensive states.
4. Hourly measurement of urine output via an indwelling catheter connected to a urinometer.
5. Measurement of the difference between skin and rectal temperature as a guide to cardiac output. Initially the difference will be high because of cutaneous vasoconstriction but, as the circulation improves, the skin vessels dilate and the skin temperature rises, so the gradient between the two temperatures falls.
6. Measurement of the acid–base state and gas tensions of arterial blood. Many samples may be needed and an arterial pressure cannula provides a convenient sampling point.
7. Regular determination of blood urea, electrolytes, haemoglobin, haematocrit, white cell and platelet counts.

Other biochemical investigations will have particular relevance in specific conditions.

In suspected bacteraemic shock two or three blood cultures and swabs or specimens from infected sites must be sent for Gram staining and bacterial culture in an attempt to identify the offending organisms.

Specific management

Hypoxia due to ventilation perfusion anomalies in the lungs is invariably present in all shocked patients. Oxygen should be accurately administered in concentrations sufficient to maintain an arterial P_{O_2} between 60 and 100 mmHg (8 and 13.3 kPa).

Hypovolaemic shock

The object is to restore a normal circulating blood volume by the administration of intravenous fluids. Virtually all cases will respond to volume replacement if it is given early enough.

The type of fluid required depends on the kind that has been lost and may therefore be whole blood, plasma, saline, dextrose (water) or any combination of these. The quantity needed is judged from the clinical state of the patient and the values of the various cardiovascular measurements; the level of the central venous pressure is particularly useful. In general, transfusion of fluid is continued until this and the other indices have returned to normal. The haematocrit is a helpful guide to plasma requirements in burnt patients and the water needs of dehydrated patients.

In many instances large volumes of fluid may have to be given rapidly and they should always be warmed to 35°C before or during infusion.

When blood is the fluid of choice but is not immediately available, a number of substitutes can be given for a limited period. These include plasma protein solutions (which are very expensive) various molecular weight dextrans, starches and certain gelatin solutions. All of them are loosely referred to as 'plasma expanders' because the size and nature of their molecular composition keeps them within the circulation for a relatively long period. Saline can be used but, since it does not stay wholly in the circulation, larger volumes are needed.

The metabolic acidosis is usually corrected by improving the circulation, and only if a severe degree persists is sodium bicarbonate required.

Vasopressor drugs (for instance, noradrenaline) have no place in the treatment of hypovolaemic shock. They cause vasoconstriction, which, although it increases pressure, reduces blood flow and so aggravates the fundamental disorder in shock.

Problems of massive blood transfusion

When given at rates greater than 8 units in 4 hours or 15 units in 24 hours, stored blood causes a number of problems:

1. *Hypothermia*. Since blood is stored at 4°C, body temperature is lowered and, as previously mentioned, a blood warmer should be used.

2. *Coagulation disturbances*. Platelets and coagulation factors decay more rapidly then red cells in stored blood and a bleeding diathesis may develop.

3. *Microembolization*. Stored blood (and frozen dry plasma) contains fragments, platelets, fibrin, and leucocytes which form microaggregates and which are filtered out in the lungs, causing pulmo-

nary dysfunction. Blood filters with a sufficiently small filter size should be used to eliminate this risk.

4. *Hyperkalaemia*. Blood stored for two weeks has a potassium content of about 20 mmol/litre. This can be a problem especially in the presence of renal insufficiency.

5. *Hypocalcaemia* may occur as a result of calcium binding by citrate which is added to blood as an anticoagulant. Calcium gluconate given intravenously corrects it.

Cardiogenic shock

The aim of treatment is to improve cardiac function and so increase cardiac output.

Hypovolaemia is rarely a major factor in cardiogenic shock but can occasionally be significant because of diminished fluid intake, sweating and prior use of diuretics. If it does exist, fluid must be replaced under very careful control—ideally, according to the level of the pulmonary wedge pressure.

The mainstay of treatment, however, is the use of drugs that increase the force of cardiac contraction—the positive inotropic agents. These almost all act by stimulating the beta-sympathetic receptors of the heart. Isoprenaline is widely used as a continuous intravenous infusion (20–120 μg per minute) but it can cause severe tachycardia and ventricular dysrhythmias. Adrenaline (20–80 μg per minute) has a similar action but suffers the same drawbacks. More recently, two new agents—dopamine and dobutamine—have been introduced. These increase cardiac output but, unlike isoprenaline and adrenaline, they have less effect on heart rate and are less likely to cause dysrhythmias. Dopamine also improves renal blood flow by a specific renal vasodilator action. The doses are dopamine 20–200 μg/kg per minute and dobutamine 50–300 μg/kg per minute. In refractory situations these drugs can be used together in various combinations.

Digitalis glycosides are inotropic drugs but their action is comparatively slow and somewhat unpredictable in shocked patients, and their acute use should be restricted to the treatment of certain dysrhythmias.

The positive inotropic drugs all have the disadvantage of increasing myocardial oxygen consumption, and in patients suffering from an acute myocardial infarction they might increase the size of the infarct if the coronary circulation cannot meet the extra demand.

Dysrhythmias are frequent in cardiogenic shock because of the nature of the underlying heart disease. They add to the circulatory disturbance and must be readily controlled.

If all such measures prove inadequate, some benefit may be obtained by reducing the work of the heart by using vasodilator drugs such as sodium nitroprusside, phentolamine or nitroglycerine, which decrease the after-load.

Despite all treatment, cardiogenic shock—especially when due to myocardial infarction—still has a depressingly high mortality, of the order of 80 per cent. Consideration has therefore been given to mechanical forms of cardiac assistance. Intra-aortic balloon counter-pulsation is currently the most popular of these and has proved to be an effective means of temporarily improving the circulation. Long-term survival is, however, less common, probably because the cardiac damage is already extensive by the time it is instituted. Consequently, it should be used only as a supportive measure in acute myocardial infarction if some form of surgical procedure, such as revascularization by sapehnous vein bypass grafting, is contemplated. Its use after open-heart surgery to wean patients off cardiopulmonary bypass has proved more rewarding.

Pulmonary oedema, often severe, may complicate the picture of cardiogenic shock. Diuretics (frusemide 40–120 mg six-hourly) are used initially, but if they are not effective intermittent positive pressure ventilation is required.

Bacteraemic shock

Antibiotics are vital to control the infection, and surgery may be necessary to remove or drain a septic focus. Fluid replacement and, in some cases, positive inotropic drugs are required to correct the circulatory disturbance which is a combination of hypovolaemia and myocardial depression.

The choice of antibiotics is dictated by the type of infecting bacterium (see Table 14.3). Clinical circumstances may be suggestive but specific identification of the organism has to await laboratory findings. Since the antibiotics must be started early, a combination that is effective against a wide range of potential pathogens is used initially and can then be modified when the results of culture are known. It is worth re-emphasizing that all specimens for bacteriological culture must be taken before starting the antibiotics.

If intestinal organisms are the likely offenders then gentamicin or one of the other aminoglycosides should be given and metronidazole added if anerobes (usually bacteroides) are suspected. If devitalized tissue is present, there is a strong possibility of a clostridial infection and large doses of soluble penicillin should be given. Flucloxacillin is added if staphylococci are suspected.

It is important to realize that such combinations of antibiotics have potentially serious side-effects, and their use must be constantly monitored and reviewed. With gentamicin the daily measurement of peak and trough blood levels determines the effective dose and helps to minimize the risks of renal and vestibular damage. Such measurements are essential in renal failure because gentamicin and the other aminoglycosides are excreted solely by the kidneys.

Steroids in shock

These have been, and still are, used indiscriminately to treat all forms of shock. The only indication for their use at present seems to be in resistant bacteraemic shock. Large doses of methylprednisolone (30 mg/kg) or dexamethasone (5 mg/kg) are then recommended.

Complications of shock

The majority of these reflect the inadequate blood flow to various vital structures.

Respiratory failure

This can arise in all forms of shock, often appearing when the circulatory problems have ben resolved. It is now the commonest cause of death in prolonged shock. Over-transfusion, microemboli, fat emboli and oxygen toxicity have all been implicated in the development of what is referred to as 'shock-lung' or the adult respiratory distress syndrome. In this condition there is a great deal of interstitial pulmonary oedema and many alveoli are filled with fibrinous and cellular debris. If extensive, these changes lead to a marked imbalance of ventilation and perfusion and severe hypoxia.

Renal failure

The reduced renal blood flow initially causes an oliguria but if it persists it can lead to established renal failure requiring dialysis.

Disseminated intravascular coagulation (DIC)

Products of tissue damage activate the clotting system and intravascular coagulation occurs in the small vessels of many organs. The formation of these small thrombi consumes the clotting factors and platelets, and therefore somewhat paradoxically the patient develops a bleeding tendency. In clinical practice, DIC may cause excessive bleeding from wounds or puncture sites, renal failure and respiratory failure.

It is diagnosed from its effects on clotting factors: the platelet count and fibrinogen level are reduced and the prothrombin time and level of fibrin degradation products (FDPs) increased.

If the DIC is severe, the patient must be heparinized; this arrests the clotting process and enables normal levels of coagulation factors to be restored.

15
Special problems

A number of cardiovascular problems are frequently encountered in the ITU. Acute myocardial infarction, massive pulmonary embolism, pericardial tamponade and acute hypertension require special mention.

Acute myocardial infarction

There are currently more than 250 000 cases of myocardial infarction each year in Britain; the incidence has now reached epidemic proportions. Of all patients affected, some 40 per cent will die within the first weeks after the attack; a quarter of these deaths occur instantaneously (that is, within 15 minutes) and a half within the first two hours. The cause of death is usually ventricular fibrillation and sometimes ventricular rupture.

The occurrence of such a high early mortality, before admission to hospital is possible, has stimulated the development of coronary ambulance or mobile coronary care services, where skilled personnel and necessary resuscitative equipment are taken to the patient. Unfortunately, with one or two exceptions, they have had very limited success, largely because of organizational problems.

In patients who survive long enough to reach hospital, the overall mortality in hospital is between 20 and 30 per cent.

Pathology

Occlusion of a coronary artery by atheroma or thrombosis interrupts the blood supply to an area of myocardium and causes death of the heart muscle cells. The area of dead cells constitutes a myocardial infarction and its extent depends on the size of the vessel occluded. Surrounding the infarct, in the acute phase, is a zone of ischaemic but still viable heart muscle. Salvage of this will limit the size of the infarct and is one of the goals of treatment.

The effects of an acute myocardial infarction on the circulation are the result of:

1. increased 'irritability' of the heart, predisposing to the development of dysrhythmias;
2. death of heart muscle, compromising the pumping action of the heart.

Clinical features

Pain usually dominates the clinical picture. It is characteristically retrosternal, with radiation into the arms, neck or jaw, and varies in severity from mild to very severe. It may last from a few minutes to several hours and is classically described as a sensation of pressure or heaviness across the chest. Nausea, vomiting and faintness may accompany the pain.

Diagnosis

This can often be confidently made from the clinical history, particularly by the description of the chest pain. It is subsequently confirmed by the ECG and serum enzyme estimations.

ECG findings

The ECG shows Q waves, ST segment elevation and T wave inversion in those leads that correspond to the site of the infarct (Fig. 15.1).

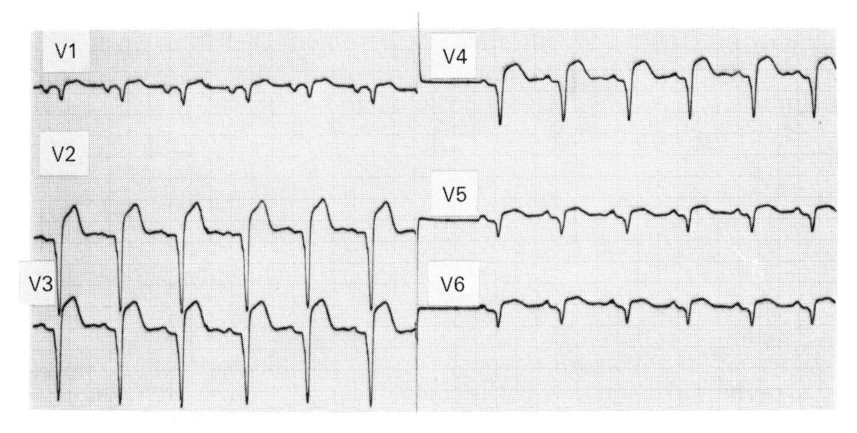

Fig. 15.1 Acute anterolateral myocardial infarction.

According to the distribution of the changes, infarcts are described as:

1. *anterior*: changes in leads V1–V3
2. *anteroseptal*: changes in leads V1–V4
3. *anterolateral*: changes in leads V1–V6
4. *inferior* changes in leads II, III, and aVF.

The ST segment elevation lasts for a few days, the T wave inversion a few weeks and the Q waves persist. Serial ECG recordings are therefore of great importance.

Serum enzymes

Heart muscle cells are rich in enzymes that are released into the circulation when the cells die. Acute damage to other tissues, such as liver and skeletal muscle, also increases certain of these enzyme levels. For the accurate diagnosis of an acute myocardial infarction it is therefore necessary to measure those enzymes that have the greatest specificity for heart muscle. These are creatine phosphokinase (CPK) and hydroxybutyric dehydrogenase (HBD).

CPK (normal level up to 60 iu/litre) is the most specific and amounts in the blood increase three or four hours after an infarction and reach a maximum level after 12–14 hours, returning to normal in 48 hours. CPK is also present in skeletal muscle, damage to which (for instance by intramuscular injections) can give misleading results.

HBD (normal level up to 300 iu/litre). This increases later than the CPK, reaching a peak level after 72 hours. It many remain elevated for several days.

Complications

There are several complications associated with acute myocardial infarction.

1. Dysrhythmias. Some form of disturbance of heart rate, rhythm or conduction is almost invariable. Many of the disturbances are transient and of little significance, whilst others precipitate major crises.

2. Cardiogenic shock develops in about 10 per cent of the cases admitted to hospital.

3. Pericarditis. If this occurs it may cause severe pain comparable to that of the original infarct but differing in that it is made worse by breathing and by lying flat.

4. Left or right ventricular failure, depending on which ventricle is predominantly affected.

5. Impaired function or rupture of the papillary muscles supporting the chordae tendineae of the mitral valve. Rupture leads to gross mitral incompetence and severe pulmonary oedema.

6. Rupture of the heart muscle, either of the ventricular wall or of the septum. The latter produces an acute ventricular septal defect.

7. Embolism. Thrombus may form on the endocardium overlying the infarct or in the left atrium if prolonged atrial fibrillation is present. Dislodgement of the thrombus produces an embolus which may occlude a systemic artery, usually cerebral, femoral or mesenteric.

There is also a high risk of deep vein thrombosis developing which can result in a pulmonary embolus.

Management

All patients with an acute myocardial infarction should, if possible, be rapidly admitted to a coronary or intensive therapy unit. The majority of problems arise in the early stages, and after 48 hours have elapsed the risk of complications falls significantly. During this first 48 hours all cases require continuous ECG monitoring and a slow intravenous infusion in case rapid administration of intravenous drugs is needed. It is necessary to emphasize that transport of the patient from the accident and emergency department to the unit should be done as quickly as possible. The ECG must be monitored during transit and resuscitation equipment kept close at hand.

The three goals of treatment are:

1. To relieve pain and control anxiety.
2. To prevent extension of the infarct and encourage healing.
3. To treat any complications promptly, as and when they arise.

The following four measures ensure the patient's comfort, reduce autonomic nervous activity, minimize the oxygen demands of the heart and so diminish the likelihood of the infarct extending.

1. *Relief of pain* is of utmost importance and usually requires diamorphine (2.5–5 mg iv) or morphine (10–15 mg iv or im) in repeated doses. Remember that blood must be taken for serum enzyme estimations before any intramusclular injection is given.

2. *Relief of anxiety* is necessary in all patients. They will require constant reassurance, explanation and nursing in a quiet environment. Diazepam (5 mg eight-hourly) should be given routinely for 48 hours.

3. *Rest.* Bed rest is necessary for the first 48 hours. Thereafter, unless complications are present, the patient should be mobilized. Uncomplicated cases are permitted to feed and shave themselves from the first day and should be allowed to use a bedside commode (which is far less 'hazardous' than a bedpan).

4. *Oxygen* is given according to the level of the arterial P_{O_2}.

The treatment of dysrhythmias and cardiogenic shock is described in Chapter 12 and Chapter 14 respectively.

Anticoagulants do not appear to influence the coronary occlusion, but in patients who cannot be mobilized quickly or who have large infarcts they reduce the risk of deep vein thrombosis and mural thrombi.

Surgery has little place in the acute attack. Papillary muscle rupture and ventricular septal defects are specific indications for repair but carry a high mortality.

Pericardial tamponade

This is a state of compression of the heart, resulting from an increase in pressure in the pericardial sac. The rise in pressure is attributable to an accumulation of fluid—blood, inflammatory exudate, pus or lymph—in the sac.

As the intrapericardial pressure increases, the heart is progressively compressed, ventricular filling is restricted, the cardiac output falls (often precipitously) and the central venous pressure rises. The speed with which these changes develop is related to the rate of rise of pressure within the pericardial sac.

The causes of pericardial tamponade are given in Table 15.1.

Table 15.1 Causes of pericardial tamponade

Type of fluid	Cause
Blood	Following cardiac surgery Chest injuries: penetrating and non-penetrating Cardiac rupture due to infarction Dissecting aneurysm Associated with anticoagulants
Inflammatory exudate and pus	Pericarditis of viral and bacterial aetiology Involvement of the pericardium by inflammatory and neoplastic disease in adjacent structures
Intravenous fluids	Perforation by a central venous line used for fluid administration

Recognition of tamponade

A constant high level of awareness is essential. The features can appear with alarming rapidity or they may develop more gradually:

1. Signs of a low cardiac output, notably tachycardia and hypotension.
2. A high central venous pressure.
3. Marked pulsus paradoxus; that is, a fall in the volume, or absence, of the pulse during inspiration. It is also recognizable, and

can be measured, by an inspiratory drop in systolic blood pressure of greater than 15 mmHg.

4. If a pericardial drain is *in situ*, as after cardiac surgery, the appearance of the clinical signs of tamponade is often associated with a reduction in pericardial drainage because the tube is obstructed.

5. Alternans of the ECG; that is, noticeable decrease in the voltage during inspiration.

Management

Treatment must be instituted quickly and the pericardial contents evacuated by either needle paracentesis or surgical drainage.

For the former, a large-bore needle is introduced beneath the xiphoid process into the pericardial sac. If fluid is collecting rapidly or is too viscous to remove through a needle then surgical drainage via a subcostal or intercostal route will be needed.

Massive pulmonary embolism

Pulmonary embolism is a common condition that, in the majority of cases, originates from venous thrombosis in the lower limbs and pelvis. The disorders which predispose to pulmonary embolism are those which cause venous thrombosis.

Its clinical presentations are varied and range from pleuritic chest pain with haemoptysis and no haemodynamic disturbance, to sudden catastrophic circulatory failure including cardiac arrest. Those patients in whom there is some degree of haemodynamic disturbance suffer from what has been termed massive pulmonary embolism and are usually treated in an ITU. When circulatory failure occurs, at least 50 per cent of the pulmonary arterial tree has been obstructed and the effects are most profound when the embolus lodges at the bifurcation of the main pulmonary artery.

Clinical features

Chest pain is comparable to that of acute myocardial infarction and is probably due to a reduction in coronary blood flow.

Syncope is present because of the lowered cerebral blood flow.

Dyspnoea may occasionally be the only symptom.

Examination of the patient reveals tachypnoea, the signs of a low cardiac output and right ventricular strain.

Investigations

The ECG is often abnormal but the changes may be delayed or transient. A normal ECG does not exclude the diagnosis.

Evidence of right heart strain often with RBBB and T wave inversion in the precordial leads are the usual changes.

Chest x-ray is most helpful for excluding other possible diagnoses such as lung collapse. The specific features of massive pulmonary embolism are not particularly striking. There may reduced vascular markings in the lung fields and dilatation of the main pulmonary artery.

Arterial blood gases show a low P_{O_2} and a low P_{CO_2} as a consequence of the hyperventilation.

Pulmonary angiography with contrast medium injected into the main pulmonary artery is the definitive investigation and should be carried out as an emergency. Emboli show as filling defects in the pulmonary arterial tree (Fig. 15.2).

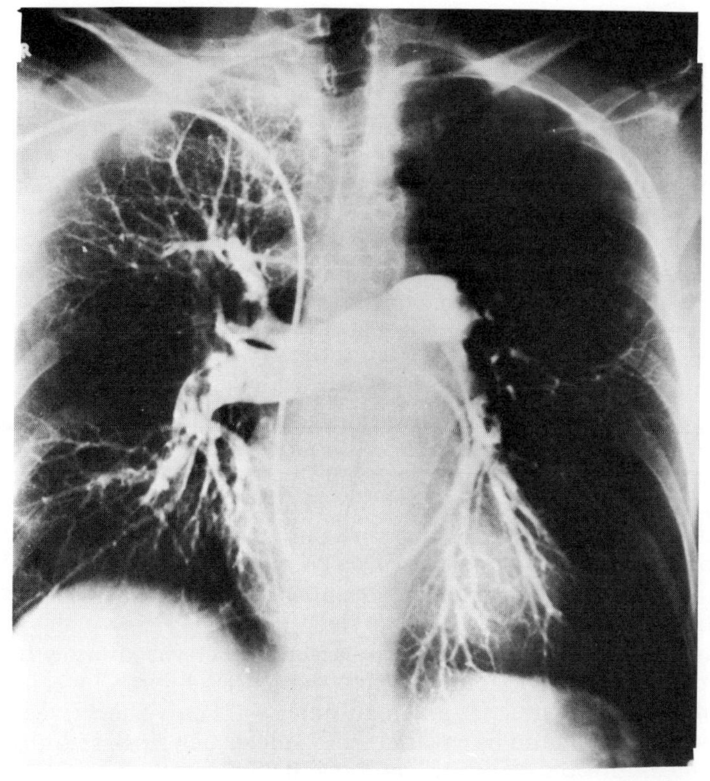

Fig. 15.2 Pulmonary angiogram showing obstruction of the left pulmonary artery.

Management

Management depends on the severity of the haemodynamic disturbance.

1. Patients with cardiac arrest require resuscitation; if an effective circulation cannot be restored, immediate embolectomy offers the only chance of saving the patient's life.

2. Patients presenting with the signs of low cardiac output should be treated with thrombolytic therapy, or anticoagulated with heparin. Streptokinase (a thrombolytic agent) in a dose of 250 000 units immediately and then 100 000 units per hour for 48–72 hours, controlled by coagulation studies, is preferred to heparin in this group. Failure to improve on this regimen is an indication for embolectomy on cardiopulmonary bypass.

3. Patients who are not shocked are anticoagulated by a continuous intravenous infusion of heparin. Oral anticoagulants are started after three to five days and continued for a minimum of three months.

Acute hypertension

Severe elevation of the arterial blood pressure may cause a variety of clinical emergencies, including hypertensive encephalopathy, left ventricular failure, intracranial haemorrhage and dissection of the aorta.

All such hypertensive emergencies require reduction of the blood pressure; in particular, those associated with acute encephalopathy or aortic dissection require immediate treatment.

Whilst there is no single level of blood pressure that produces a hypertensive crisis, the majority of cases will have a diastolic pressure of between 110 and 150 mmHg. Irrespective of the cause, patients with hypertensive emergencies are admitted to the ITU for lowering and control of their arterial pressure. A variety of drugs are available and their administration should be carefully controlled by continuous direct monitoring of the arterial pressure. Often in the early stages of treatment the levels of blood pressure oscillate and frequent adjustment of dosage may be necessary. Treatment is easier to control using drugs that can be given by continuous intravenous infusion and which have a short duration of action.

1. *Sodium nitroprusside* is a rapidly acting direct vasodilator. It has a short duration of action and must therefore be given by continuous infusion. If too much is given, the effects are only short lived. The infusion bottle should be covered with a paper bag since sodium nitroprusside is affected by light. The dose is 0.05–0.2 mg per minute. Sodium nitroprusside is converted in the body to thiocyanate, and

with infusions of longer than 72 hours mental confusion and other neurological symptoms may develop. Thiocyanate levels in the blood should be measured with long-term therapy.

2. *Diazoxide* is a non-diuretic thiazide and exerts a hypotensive effect by dilatation of the arteries. When given intravenously its effects may persist for 12 hours or longer. The dose is 300 mg intravenously once or twice daily.

3. *Hydrallazine* is especially effective in hypertensive crises associated with renal disease. The dose is 10–20 mg intravenously immediately, followed by 10–50 mg intramuscularly four- to six-hourly. It can also be given by continuous intravenous infusion.

4. *Phentolamine* is an alpha-adrenergic blocking agent. It has a short duration of action and, like sodium nitroprusside, is given by continuous intravenous infusion. It is particular value in the hypertensive crises associated with phaeochromocytomas. The dose is 5–15 mg immediately, followed by 0.5–1 mg per minute.

Other drugs may be used from time to time, including reserpine, methyldopa, diuretics and various beta blockers.

16
Nursing care

Nursing care of the cardiovascular system is always a significant part of the total nursing care but in certain cases it is the dominant aspect; for example, in patients suffering from an acute myocardial infarction or recovering from cardiac surgery.

In caring for such patients there are many inter-related nursing techniques which, for convenience, are divided into (1) the management of monitoring equipment, (2) the details of certain specific procedures and (3) the nursing practice during cardiac arrest and resuscitation.

Nursing management of monitoring equipment

This includes the care and use of electrocardiographic, vascular pressure and temperature monitoring equipment.

ECG monitoring

Disposable, adhesive electrodes are used, three of which are usually positioned on the chest (Fig. 16.1) avoiding, if possible, sites that are directly over muscles since this helps to decrease artefacts from muscle tremor. Initially some alteration of position may be necessary to obtain a clear ECG waveform. In the presence of extensive chest dressing, limb electrodes will be needed. Careful skin preparation and firm attachment of the electrodes are essential, for the skin–electrode junction is the main source of interference. To achieve good contact, it is necessary to:

1. Shave the sites of placement.
2. Rub the skin with gauze soaked in a spirit base solution to remove the skin's natural oils.
3. Allow the skin to dry.
4. Prepare the electrodes by applying, if necessary, conductive gel and removing the protective backings.

5. Position and secure the electrodes in place by applying firm pressure to the adhesive portions.

The electrodes can now be connected to the three, colour-coded, terminals of the patient cable, labelled left arm, right arm and left leg. By convention, the right arm terminal is connected to the electrode on the upper right side of the chest, the left arm terminal to the one on the upper left side and the left leg terminal to the inferior electrode. However, this may not always be the most satisfactory arrangement and changing the terminals from one electrode to another may produce a larger and clearer ECG waveform.

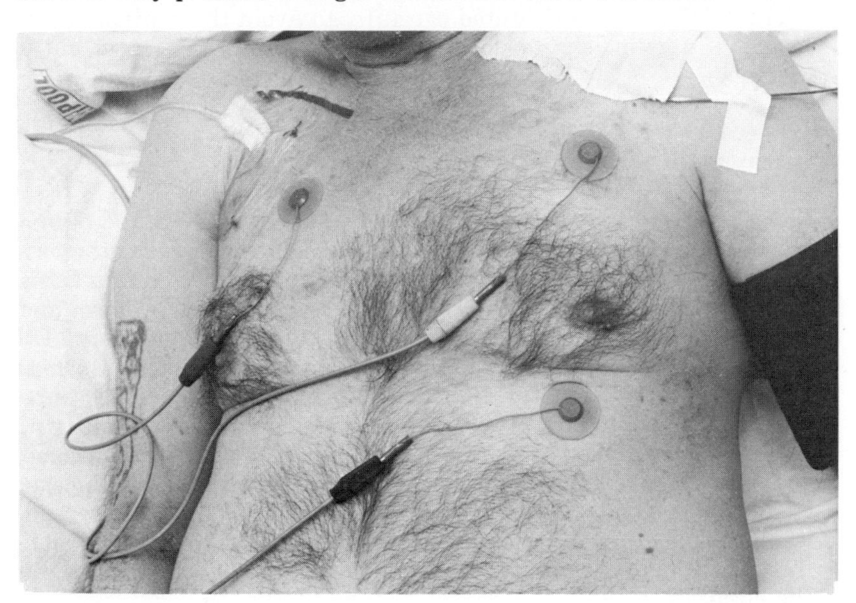

Fig. 16.1 Electrode positions.

Replacement of one or all the electrodes is necessary if:

1. The electrode becomes loose and cannot be refixed. (This may occur if the conductive gel has spilled onto the adhesive ring, or when the patient is restless or perspiring.) To improve electrode fixation in restless or perspiring patients, adhesive plaster or micropore strips can be placed over the electrodes.

2. There is skin irritation around the electrode site.

3. There is still 'interference' on the monitor and all other causes of this have been eliminated.

Each time an electrode is changed, the skin preparation must be repeated and any dried gel removed.

In addition to looking after the ECG monitoring, the nurse may be required, from time to time, to record a 12-lead ECG. For this, metal plate limb electrodes with sockets into which the patient's cable is secured are used. They are fixed in position with rubber bands. Before applying the plates, the nurse must check that they are clean and free of dried electrode gel. A liberal amount of conduction gel is placed on the plates and one is positioned on each limb, just above the wrist and ankle, again avoiding the muscle and hair areas. The cable is connected; each of its terminals are clearly labelled for the appropriate limb. Correct anatomical positioning of the chest electrode is extremely important. After the recording has been made, the skin areas are cleaned and the plates and rubber bands thoroughly washed and dried.

The ECG must be mounted carefully to avoid the confusion that results if part of it is upside-down, in the wrong section or out of sequence.

Intravascular catheters

These are used to record arterial, central venous (CVP) and pulmonary wedge pressure (PWP). To detect these pressures, a catheter is passed into an appropriate artery or vein and connected to a transducer which is linked to the oscilloscope where the waveform and, sometimes, the absolute values are displayed continuously. The patency of the catheter is maintained by a continuous 'flushing device' between it and the transducer. This device, which the nurse must know how to use, provides a means of 'flushing' the line (with either 5 per cent dextrose or normal saline) when the trace becomes damped. On occasions the catheter may become completely blocked by a clot of blood. A syringe can be attached to the catheter and withdrawal of the blood clot attempted, but on no account should it be flushed through the vessel because of the danger of dispersing it into the circulation.

Care is essential in handling the transducer; it is a delicate and expensive piece of equipment and its calibration is the responsibility of the medical or technical staff.

The reference level

All measurements must be recorded from a definite zero level because placing the transducer at different levels relative to the patient alters the reading. For all three measurements—arterial, central venous and pulmonary wedge pressure—common reference points are the sternal angle and mid-axillary line (fourth intercostal space). The mid-axillary line is preferred because it is anatomically in line with the right atrium.

The transducer is either fixed in position with plaster (Fig. 16.2a) or mounted on a table and the height of the transducer table adjusted to the zero reference level. Accurate alignment is achieved by using a spirit level fixed in a wooden or telescopic arm; it is easier if the point on the patient is marked (Fig. 16.2b). Each time the recording is made, the position of the transducer must be checked because the patient's position or the height of the bed may have changed since the previous reading.

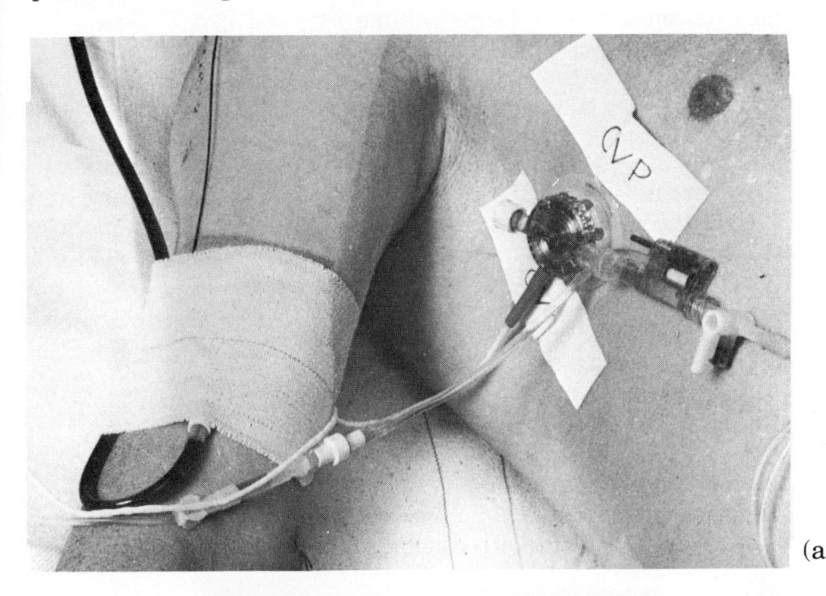

(a)

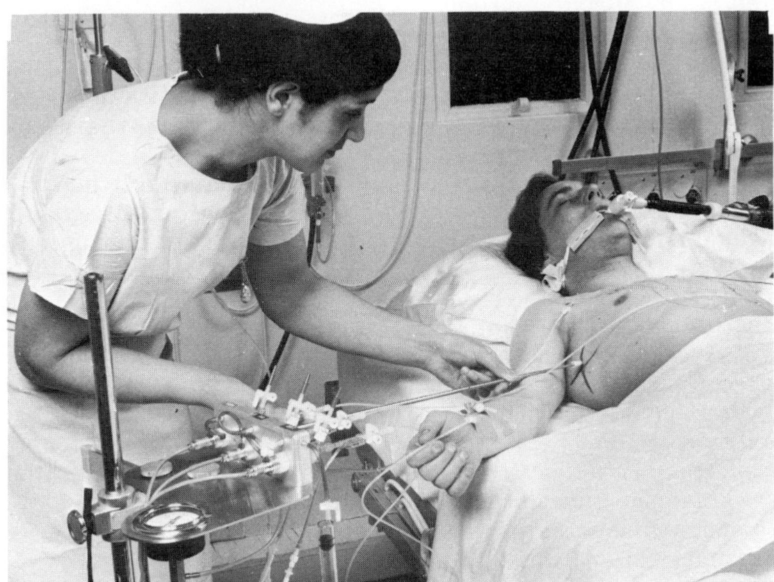

(b)

Fig. 16.2 (a) Transducer fixed in position by adhesive plaster. (b) Use of a telescopic arm to align transducer table to reference level (X).

Care of an arterial catheter
The nurse must ensure that the catheter is not under any tension, not kinked and firmly connected to the pressure line. If the catheter becomes disconnected, a large volume of blood can be lost very quickly.

Frequently the radial artery is cannulated; the ideal splint for protecting the arm is a light-weight one that leaves exposed the insertion point of the catheter, its connection and the forearm. The area is checked regularly for signs of local infection, evidence of impaired circulation in the territory supplied by the artery and bleeding at the point of insertion of the catheter. Obstruction of the local arterial circulation causes blanching and mottling and a fall in skin temperature.

Drugs should never be given through an arterial line, and usually the catheter is not left *in situ* for longer than 48 or 72 hours. On its removal, firm pressure is applied over the puncture site for a minimum of five minutes to prevent haematoma formation; a sterile dressing is then placed firmly over the area.

Care of a central venous catheter
This is based on similar principles. Complications of central venous catheterization can arise both during and after its insertion.

Complications during insertion
Two particular complications can occur during insertion.

1. Using the subclavian or internal jugular veins, air embolism may occur if the patient is not placed in a head-down position. Such a position ensures a positive venous pressure and eliminates the risk of 'sucking' air into the veins.
2. Neighbouring anatomical structures may be damaged when the subclavian vein is cannulated: the pleura may be penetrated, causing a pneumothorax, or the subclavian artery damaged, resulting in a haemothorax.

Complications after insertion
Any of several complications may arise after the catheter has been inserted.

1. Blockage due to kinking of the catheter or obstruction of its lumen by a blood clot.
2. Infection, either locally around the catheter site or systemically due to organisms introduced through the catheter.
3. Venous thrombosis, particularly if the line is used for infusion of hypertonic solutions which are highly irritant.
4. Pericardial tamponade due to the catheter piercing the wall of the right atrium and entering the pericardial sac.

The catheter may have to be left *in situ* for several days or even weeks. Sterility is therefore essential when handling any item connected to the catheter or the catheter itself. The dressing over the point of insertion must be changed daily and the site inspected for signs of infection. Use of a transparent dressing makes this unnecessary. In the event of infection or evidence of bacteraemia, the same principles apply as detailed in Chapter 10.

A fluid manometer is commonly used for measuring central venous pressure. This consists of a measuring column mounted on a centimetre scale and connected to an intravenous giving set via a three-way tap. The manometer can be attached to a ruler and held against the reference point (Fig. 16.3). Otherwise, a spirit level in a wooden or telescopic arm is required. The same zero reference levels are used as for measurement made with a transducer. In both instances alignment must be accurate because CVP is a low pressure and small errors result in significant errors of its true value. To measure the CVP with a fluid manometer:

1. Place the patient flat, or, if for some reason this is not possible, at an angle of 45°. All subsequent recordings must be taken in this original position.

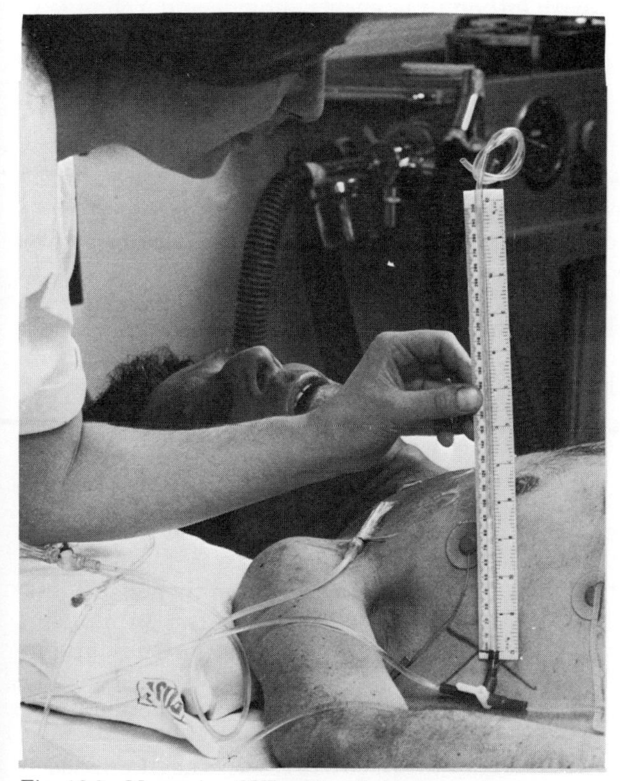

Fig. 16.3 Measuring CVP with a fluid manometer.

2. Allow the infusion (either 5 per cent dextrose or normal saline) to run freely for a few seconds to flush the catheter and ensure its patency.
3. Turn the three-way tap to allow fluid to run into the measuring column.
4. Establish the zero reference level with the indicator.
5. Turn the three-way tap to connect the measuring column to the catheter.
6. Read the value of the CVP once the fluid level has stabilized; it fluctuates with respiration.
7. Turn the three-way tap to connect the catheter and the infusion, and adjust the drip rate to run slowly to maintain the patency of the catheter.

Care of a flotation catheter

The problems of blockage and infection apply equally to these catheters but with care they can be left in place for three days without causing complications.

To obtain a recording, alignment of the zero reference is checked, the balloon inflated with either air or carbon dioxide and a change is seen in the pressure tracing denoting the PWP. The prescribed inflation volume should never be exceeded because of the dangers of balloon rupture. In between measurements the balloon is left deflated.

Care of a pacemaker

This requires the nurse to confirm that the system is functioning correctly and, according to instruction, whether it is in a demand or continuous pacing mode. The nurse must verify from the monitor and by counting the patient's pulse rate that pacing is maintained at the desired rate. Routine checks are made to ensure that the connections between the pacemaker box and the leads are satisfactory. The insertion site of the catheter is dressed aseptically daily and inspected for signs of infection.

Temperature recording

Temperature may be measured electronically using thermistor probes; when continuous records are necessary, as for example in hypothermic states, this method is less disturbing for the patient. Central body (core) temperature is monitored by a probe inserted into the rectum, and skin (peripheral) temperature by attachment of a probe to a big toe.

Rectal probes have a tendency to fall out; to reduce the likelihood of this happening, the cable from the probe must be securely fixed to the buttock or thigh with either micropore tape or adhesive plaster. The skin probe is placed on a great toe, covered with a piece of cotton wool and fixed in position with plaster; if left exposed, it will measure the room, rather than the skin, temperature. If a sudden change of temperature occurs in either the central or skin temperature between recordings the nurse must check the position of the appropriate probe.

When several functions are being monitored, to avoid tangling the equipment the various lines and cables should be arranged separately for easy identification and the transducers clearly labelled (Fig. 16.4). The alarm devices warn the nurse that something is amiss. Some of the alarms will be false ones arising from improper use of the

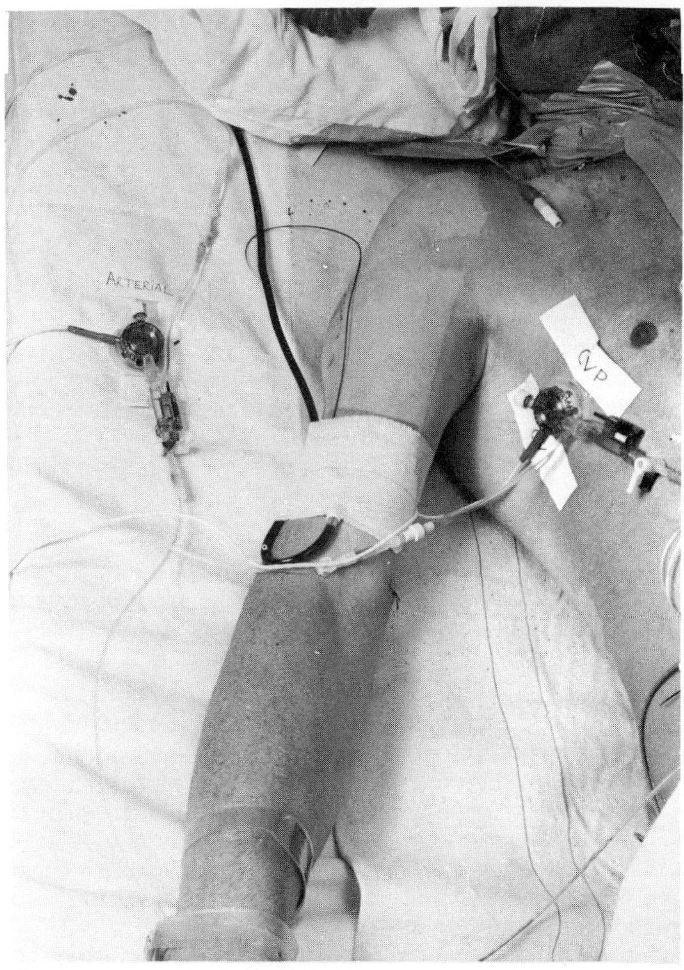

Fig. 16.4 Pressure transducers; labelled to avoid confusion.

equipment or misplacement of an electrode or transducer. The nurse's first action on hearing an alarm must be to look at the patient, quickly assessing the clinical condition, and then to check the equipment.

Nursing procedures in specific conditions

Acute myocardial infarction

These patients are often extremely anxious and in severe pain. They are normally alert and aware of the nature of their illness and their anxiety and fear have adverse effects, causing tachycardia and sometimes dysrhythmias. The anxiety if often accentuated by the special natue of the unit and it is most important that on arrival the patient be greeted by a calm, confident, reassuring nurse, who explains the function of the unit. Emphasis should not be placed on the monitoring equipment because this may increase the patient's agitation.

Procedures on admission

Upon admission to the unit, the nurse should:

1. Position the patient comfortably and give oxygen via a facemask.
2. Establish continuous ECG monitoring and observe the rhythm and rate of the heart.
3. Record the pulse rate, apex rate, blood pressure, respiratory rate and temperature. The frequency of subsequent measurements will be dictated by the patient's clinical condition.
4. Relieve the patient's pain and nausea according to medical instructions.
5. Record a 12-lead ECG.

The medical staff will set up an intravenous infusion to facilitate the administration of drugs and to save time in the event of serious dysrhythmias or cardiac arrest.

General nursing care

The patient requires all the nursing care of any patient who is confined to bed, but routines must be flexible to allow maximum rest. For the conscious patient the sitting position is usually most comfortable and allows better expansion of the lung bases. Measurement of the arterial P_{O_2} will determine the need for oxygen therapy. A light diet and fluids are permitted and an accurate fluid balance chart must be kept. Whenever possible, the patient is allowed to use a bedside commode which imposes less strain than using a bedpan; laxatives may help with this aspect of care. Pain is a source of distress to the patient and must be controlled promptly. A combination of an analgesic and a sedative are often most beneficial. Passive limb exercises, to prevent a deep vein thrombosis developing, are carried out several times a day and the patient is encouraged to move, particularly his legs, at intervals.

A great part of the nurse's duty is devoted to watching the ECG. In a coronary care unit this is usually done by one nurse at a central console. This duty, because it requires sustained concentration, should be relieved regularly. In addition, the patient is observed regularly for signs of cyanosis, dyspnoea, cold extremities and altered consciousness, all of which are indicators of a failing cardiac output.

Patients who have had a myocardial infarction require a considerable amount of psychological support and encouragement from both nursing and medical staff. They are often aware of the risk of sudden death and are apprehensive about the future. Their distress can be increased if they are aware of activities in other bed areas, so nursing in separate rooms is essential to ensure a quiet and calm atmosphere.

The most crucial period after a myocardial infarction is the first 48 hours because of the high risk of complications. Transfer to a general ward is considered after this period if the patient is free from acute problems.

Cardiac surgery

Cardiac surgery is carried out on patients with coronary artery disease, those with acquired valve disease and patients with congenital lesions. However, regardless of the specific nature of the operation the immediate postoperative nursing care follows a similar pattern.

Preparing the bed area for reception of the patient

This is done while the operation is in progress. It is set up in the usual manner but with certain additional items: 'milking' rollers for the chest drains, and emergency drugs (adrenaline, isoprenaline and calcium chloride) which are checked, drawn up into syringes and clearly labelled.

The bed is taken to the operating theatre with an intravenous infusion stand, a portable oxygen cylinder, oxygen tubing, a Waters' canister (rebreathing bag), a holder for the chest drainage bottles and two pairs of clamps for the chest drains.

During transfer to the unit, the ECG and the arterial pressure are monitored on a portable oscilloscope and the patient is hand ventilated.

Initial procedures on the patient's arrival in the unit

The following procedures are carried out as soon as the patient arrives in the unit.

1. Establish ventilation.

2. Establish ECG monitoring.

3. Establish pressure monitoring from the intravascular catheters and check for any oozing of blood from the insertion sites since, if present, this may indicate coagulation problems.

4. Unclamp the chest drains and attach them to suction. Record the level of drainage in each underwater seal bottle and also check for any oozing of blood from around each drain site.

5. Check the flow rates of the individual infusions.

6. Insert the thermistor probe into the rectum and attach the peripheral probe to a toe.

7. Ensure that the urinary catheter is attached to a calibrated drainage bag.

8. Observe the patient, noting in particular skin colour, level of consciousness and degree of comfort.

9. Start recording and charting observations.

10. Secure the nasogastric tube drainage bag, if present, to the bed. A nasogastric tube is generally *in situ* to prevent distension of the stomach and consequent respiratory embarrassment.

11. Check the pacing wires, if present.

In order to accomplish these procedures quickly it is necessary for two nurses to receive the patient, both then remaining at the bedside until the patient is settled and his condition is stable. Having completed these steps the subsequent management is dictated by the patient's progress.

Records

Recordings are made of:

1. Heart rate and rhythm.
2. Pulse rate.
3. Arterial pressure.
4. Central venous pressure; left atrial pressure.
5. Core and peripheral temperatures
6. Ventilation.
7. Urine volume.
8. Intravenous fluid replacement of blood or other colloids and crystalloid infusions.
9. Volume of blood loss from each chest drain.
10. Nasogastric drainage.

In addition, the patient is observed continuously to determine his colour, degree of comfort and level of consciousness.

Care of the chest drains

Drains are routinely inserted into the mediastinum and into the pericardium. If the pleural cavity has been opened at surgery then a third drain will have been inserted into the pleura. Each drain is connected to a calibrated underwater seal bottle, with the level of the water in the bottle clearly marked. The drain is attached to the long tube under the water level and suction applied to the shorter tube. The drains are connected to the same suction unit via a Y piece (Fig. 16.5). Suction may be applied either from a Robert's sucker or a wall suction unit. The drainage tubes and volume of drainage must be constantly checked and the tubes 'milked' hourly with rollers to prevent blockage. The frequency of 'milking' is increased if blood clots are seen in the drainage. Great care is needed when moving the patient to avoid disconnecting the drains and allowing air to enter the chest. To prevent this the drains are clamped prior to movement.

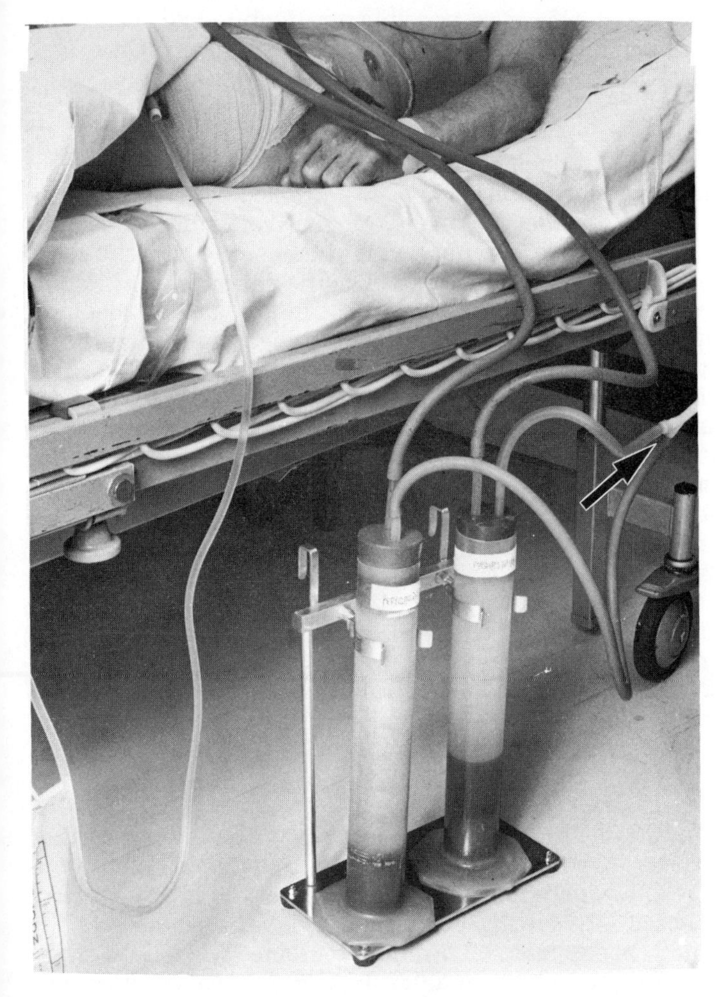

Fig. 16.5 Mediastinal (right) and pericardial (left) drains (the Y connection (arrow) is attached to the suction apparatus).

The chest drains are removed when the drainage has ceased or is minimal—usually the day after operation. The pericardial drain is removed first, leaving the mediastinal one *in situ* in case the removal of the first drain causes some bleeding. Once it is certain that there is no increase in the amount of drainage, the mediastinal drain is removed.

Removing a chest drain is an aseptic procedure. Both intrathoracic and intrapleural drains must be removed quickly to prevent the introduction of air into either cavity. Frequently a 'purse-string' suture will have been used to secure the drain in position. In order to remove the drain quickly and minimize the risk of air entry, two nurses are required. One is responsible for dividing and then tying the suture while the other nurse withdraws the drain. Once it is removed, a sterile dressing is applied over the site.

Complications

Excessive bleeding is not always apparent as an increase in the chest drainage volume because it may be concealed. When bleeding is concealed, the patient develops signs of hypovolaemia out of proportion to the quantity of drainage. Slight adjustments of the chest drains and 'milking' the tubing may be sufficient to produce drainage. Replacement of blood by transfusion can at times be adequate but continuous bleeding will require the patient to return to the operating theatre.

Pericardial tamponade is an acute collection of blood in the pericardium. It usually develops during the first 24 hours after surgery, although it can occasionally be a later complication. The accumulation of blood in the pericardium restricts cardiac filling and the cardiac output falls. The signs of tamponade are therefore:

1. A reduced pericardial drainage.
2. A falling blood pressure.
3. A rising pulse rate.
4. A rising CVP measurement.
5. A decreasing urinary output.

A chest x-ray may show an increase in the size of the heart shadow. Surgical exploration is essential unless prompt, adequate pericardial drainage can be achieved by manupulation of the drain.

General nursing care

The sitting position is the optimum position for nursing postcardiac surgical patients. In this posture, pericardial and mediastinal drainage is assisted and there is better ventilation of the lungs, particularly their bases. The sitting position is gradually adopted as the patient's condition becomes stable, and is combined with slight elevation of the foot of the bed which helps to promote venous return and also prevents the patient sliding down the bed. Passive limb movements are given, particularly leg excercises, to reduce the incidence of a deep vein thrombosis. When leg veins have been removed for coronary artery bypass grafting, the incisions are checked frequently for oozing of blood. If this is present, local pressure is usually sufficient to control it.

The chest dressing is taken down for inspection the morning after operation and redressed aseptically. If the immediate postoperative phase has been uncomplicated, the patient is transferred to a ward 24–48 hours after surgery.

Cardiac arrest

The initial stages of resuscitation are usually started by the nurse who is caring for that particular patient. She summons help by ringing the 'cardiac arrest' bell, lies the patient flat, ensures a clear airway and institutes external cardiac massage and assisted ventilation. The speed at which these maneouvres are begun and their effectiveness are crucial.

When a cardiac arrest occurs in the unit, the immediate nursing priorities must be to:

1. Inform the medical staff.
2. Relieve the nurse at the bedside of both external cardiac massage and assisted ventilation by allocating another nurse.
3. Collect and bring to the bed area the resuscitation and intubation trolley.
4. Prepare, in syringes, the appropriate drugs—sticking the ampoules onto the syringes with transparent tape (Sellotape) to avoid errors.
5. Prepare the defibrillator by applying conductive gel to the paddles and charging the machine.

Formal documentation of the drugs given and the number and strength of d.c. shocks is important.

Resuscitation can be a long and somewhat complicated procedure; to avoid any confusion concerning responsibilities, the senior nurse present should co-ordinate the activities of the nursing staff.

Resuscitation equipment

The resuscitation trolley should be compact in design and freely mobile. The daily checking of the contents and the priming and discharging of the defibrillator current must be routine policy, and is the responsibility of either the technical or the senior nursing staff. The trolley must contain:

1. A defibrillator and paddles.
2. Conductive gel.
3. An ECG writer if this is not included in the bedside monitor.
4. Five per cent dextrose.
5. Sodium bicarbonate (8.4 per cent solution).
6. Standard intravenous infusion sets.
7. Burette-type intravenous sets.

8. A selection of drugs:

Adrenaline
Aminophylline
Atropine
Calcium chloride
Calcium gluconate
Dexamethasone
Diazepam
Frusemide
Hydrocortisone
Isoprenaline
Lignocaine
Potassium chloride
Practolol
Procainamide

Other necessary items of equipment are: cardiac pacemakers, a bronchoscopy set and a sterile thoracotomy set.

Section D
Respiratory failure

17
Acute respiratory failure

Definition

Respiratory failure is now defined in relation to abnormal arterial blood gas tensions: P_{O_2} of less than 60 mmHg (8 kPa) or a P_{CO_2} greater than 49 mmHg (6.5 kPa) values that are well outside the normal physiological range.

Classification

In accordance with this definition, respiratory failure is classified into:

1. Hypoxaemic (low P_{O_2}).
2. Ventilatory (high P_{CO_2}).
3. A combination of 1 and 2 (low P_{O_2} and a high P_{CO_2}).

It is necessary to make a clear distinction between acute and chronic respiratory failure. The former develops quickly in previously healthy lungs whilst the latter progresses slowly over a period of years. Acute-on-chronic failure is due to an acute respiratory insult inflicted on lungs that are already damaged.

Hypoxaemic failure

Hypoxaemic failure is caused by acute diseases affecting the lung tissue (Table 17.1). Pathologically, the lung reacts in a similar manner to a variety of acute infections and toxins. There is an inflammatory cell reaction with oedema and the alveoli become filled with exudate and fibrinous material. Not surprisingly therefore, the clinical picture of acute hypoxaemic respiratory failure is rather nonspecific and, in the past, has had various names. These have included 'white lung', 'shock lung' and, more recently, 'the adult respiratory distress syndrome'.

The hypoxaemia is a consequence of ventilation/perfusion inequalities. Blood perfuses alveoli that have no, or inadequate, ventilation because they are either collapsed or contain fluid and inflammatory debris. The magnitude of this shunting or venous admixture determines the degree of hypoxaemia. The respiratory centre in the brain stem is stimulated by the hypoxaemia, causing the patient to hyperventilate; as a result it is common to find a low P_{O_2} associated with a low P_{CO_2}.

Most organs or tissues can function until the P_{O_2} falls below 30 mmHg (4 kPa) and such a degree of hypoxaemia is therefore extremely dangerous and potentially fatal, more so if the circulation is also affected.

Table 17.1 Causes of hypoxaemic respiratory failure

Specific infections	Bacterial Viral Fungal
Non-specific aggravating factors	Multiple transfusions Oxygen toxicity Disseminated intravascular coagulation (DIC)
Associated with trauma	Contusion of the lung Fat emboli
Associated with cardiac failure	Pulmonary oedema

Ventilatory failure

This occurs when the ventilatory forces are inadequate to ventilate the alveoli: the elevated P_{CO_2} signifies the hypoventilation. Effective ventilation requires a completely integrated neuromuscular mechanism; it can be affected by a variety of diseases which cause ventilatory failure (Table 17.2).

Table 17.2 Causes of ventilatory failure

Central nervous system	Head injury Drug overdose Cerebrovascular accidents Encephalitis Status epilepticus Tetanus
Cervical cord lesions	Trauma
Spinal motor neurone	Poliomyelitis
Peripheral nerve	Polyneuritis (e.g. Guillain–Barré syndrome)
Neuromuscular junction	Myasthenia gravis Muscle relaxant drugs (e.g. curare)
Chest wall and muscles	Injury—(e.g. flail segment) Deformities Myopathies

Hypoxaemic and ventilatory failure not uncommonly coexist. For example, a patient with a serious chest injury may develop 'shock lung; or one who has taken a drug overdose may inhale gastric contents and develop an aspiration pneumonia.

Clinical picture and diagnosis

The clinical manifestations of acute respiratory failure are somewhat non-specific and in the early stages they can be difficult to recognize. Diagnosis has to be qualified by measurement of the blood gas tensions.

Hypoxaemia affects the central nervous system, causing hyperventilation, restlessness, confusion and, when very severe, stupor and coma. The sympathetic nervous system is activated, producing tachycardia, hypertension and sweating. Cyanosis, best looked for in the mucous membrane of the mouth, is seen only when the hypoxaemia is severe ($P\text{O}_2$ less than 50 mmHg or 6.7 kPa).

The features of carbon dioxide retention are very variable. At high levels ($P\text{CO}_2$ greater than 80 mmHg or 10.7 kPa) it causes drowsiness, confusion and coma. With lower values there is a reversal of sleep rhythm: the patient is drowsy during the day and wide awake at night. A flapping tremor (asterixis) may be present and, because carbon dioxide is a vasodilator, the patient has warm peripheries and a bounding circulation.

Measurements of tidal volume, vital capacity and peak flow rate are helpful in assessing the state of ventilation, and repeat measurements enable the progress of the disease to be followed.

Investigations

Arterial blood gas analysis is essential to establish the severity of the respiratory failure and to monitor the effects of treatment on the course of the disease.

Chest x-ray. Portable x-ray films are of diagnostic value and can show the distribution of the underlying disease. Sequential films provide a sensitive measure of change. In ventilated patients the position of the endotracheal or tracheostomy tube can be checked.

Sputum cultures. In respiratory infections, samples of sputum are sent for microscopy, culture and sensitivity. These samples should be obtained from coughed up specimens but, if this is impossible or if the patient has an endotracheal or tracheostomy tube, they are obtained via a suction trap. In severe infections, blood cultures are necessary.

Haemoglobin and white cell counts are checked daily. Low levels of haemoglobin can have a critical effect on oxygen transport; white cell counts are of diagnostic and prognostic help.

Twelve-lead ECG. This may show dysrhythmias, right ventricular strain or right ventricular hypertrophy. The P waves may be peaked—'P pulmonale'.

Management

The essence of treatment is to correct the hypoxaemia and support ventilation whilst the primary disease is treated. Often in respiratory failure other body systems, especially the cardiovascular, are affected and detailed attention to their function is an integral part of management.

Oxygen therapy

Mild degrees of hypoxaemia do not appear to be harmful. A fall in P_{O_2} to 60 mmHg (8 kPa) causes only a 10 per cent fall in oxygen saturation. Below this level, however, on the steep part of the oxyhaemoglobin dissociation curve, oxygen content falls relatively quickly. It is appropriate to start oxygen therapy when the P_{O_2} falls to levels of between 60 and 70 mmHg (8 and 9.3 kPa).

The concentration and flow rate of the oxygen administered needs to be sufficient to maintain the P_{O_2} at around 70 mmHg (9.3 kPa); there is no physiological rationale, or clinical merit, in striving to keep it at any higher level.

Several kinds of facemasks are now available and they enable the concentration of oxygen in the inspired air to be varied over a wide range. It is, however, not possible to give 100 per cent oxygen in this way because leaks are present around even the most carefully applied and closest fitting mask. Sixty per cent is the highest concentration of oxygen that can be reliably and continuously administered to a patient who is not intubated.

In hypoxaemic failure, if the ventilation/perfusion abnormality is so great that even the maximal inspiratory concentration of oxygen (60 per cent) cannot correct the arterial P_{O_2}, the patient will very likely have to be intubated and ventilated.

In pure ventilatory failure, oxygen is not initially the dominant need but, as the ventilation decreases, coughing and sighing are impaired and sputum retention, atelectasis and infection occur; these will eventually cause hypoxaemia.

Intermittent positive pressure ventilation (IPPV)

Indications

The object of IPPV is to provide adequate ventilation (elimination of carbon dioxide) and oxygenation with minimal damage to the lungs and minimal disturbance of the circulation. It is achieved by intermittently inflating the lungs with gas under a positive pressure: the natural elastic properties of the lungs provide the necessary recoil to expel the gases (Fig. 17.1).

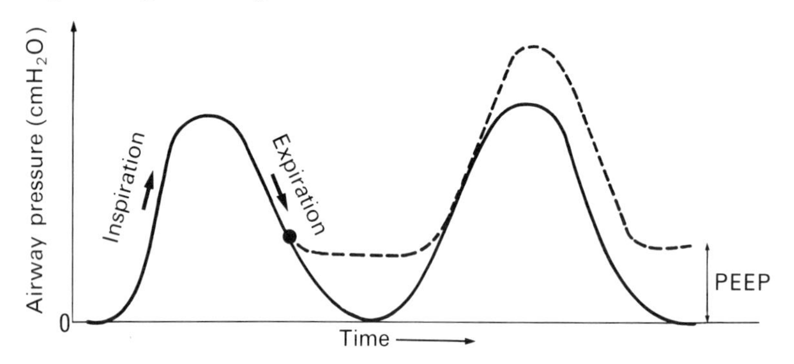

Fig. 17.1 Ventilatory pressure waveforms showing the effect of adding a PEEP.

Any system for IPPV (Fig.17.2) consists of a ventilator, inspiratory and expiratory connecting tubes, and a humidifier since all gases given to intubated patients must be humidified. The necessary pattern of ventilation is obtained by regulating the tidal volume, the respiratory frequency, the length of inspiration and expiration, and the oxygen concentration of the inspired air. It varies from patient to patient depending of the cause and severity of the respiratory failure.

Usually there is no single criterion or rule that indicates the necessity for IPPV. Hypoxia, hypercapnia, excessive secretions, fatigue and disorders in the other systems often coexist and additively contribute to the need for artificial ventilation.

In uncomplicated acute ventilatory failure, the situation can be more clearly defined with a $P\text{CO}_2$ of greater than 55 mmHg (7.3 kPa) and/or a vital capacity of less than 1 litre, providing strong indications for IPPV.

The principle guidelines for instituting ventilation in hypoxaemic and mixed respiratory failure are shown in Table 17.3.

Endotracheal intubation

This is necessary before IPPV can be started. An endotracheal tube of appropriate size is passed into the trachea (Fig. 17. 3), through either the mouth or nose; the choice of route depends on particular clinical

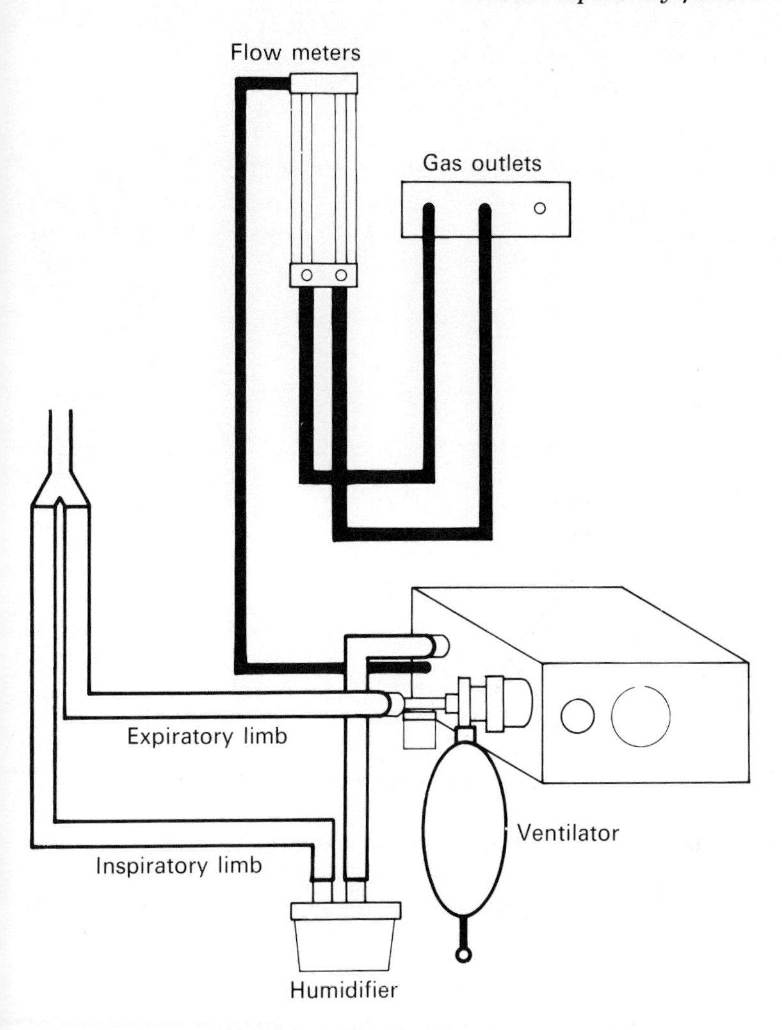

Fig. 17.2 System for IPPV.

Table 17.3 The principal indications for endotracheal intubation and ventilation

An arterial P_{O_2} of less than 60 mmHg (8 kPa) on maximal concentration of inspired oxygen
A P_{CO_2} of greater than 55 mmHg (7.3 kPa)
Protection of the airway in deeply unconscious patients
Postoperatively, where respiratory failure is anticipated; e.g. following cardiac surgery, in obese and debilitated patients with preoperative respiratory problems

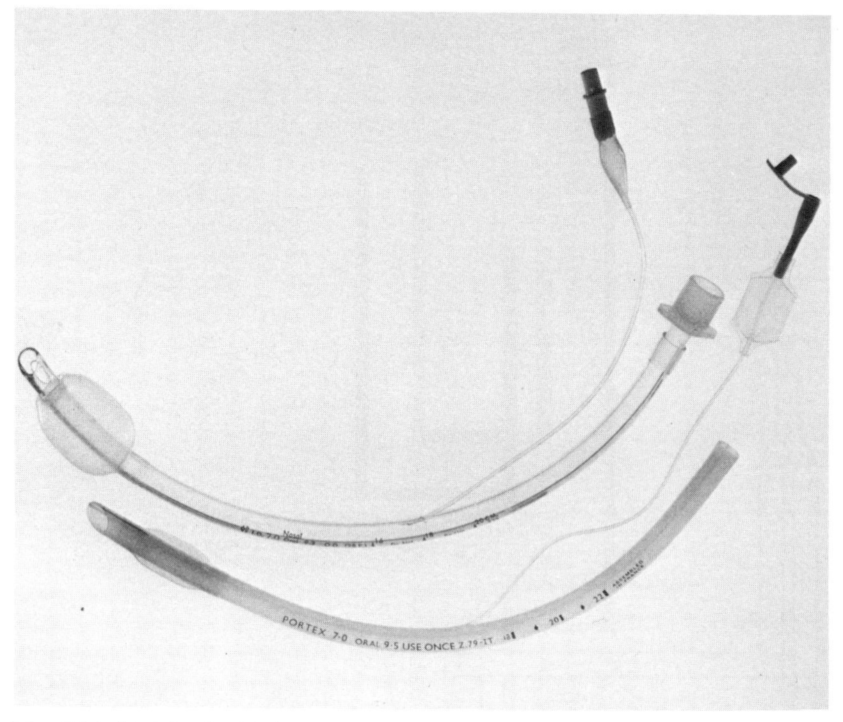

Fig. 17.3 Endotracheal tubes.

circumstances. The size of an endotracheal tube is given in millimetres, according to the internal diameter. Oral tubes range from 5.0 to 11.0 mm in 0.5 mm stages; nasal tubes, likewise, range from 5.0 to 9.0 mm.

Orotracheal intubation allows a wider and shorter tube to be used but fixing and stabilizing it after insertion is difficult and its presence in the mouth interferes with nursing care. Conscious patients find oral tubes very uncomfortable and can obstruct them by biting.

A nasal tube must be longer and narrower (the nose is the narrowest part of the airway) and therefore it has a greater tendency to kink and makes suction more difficult. It is, however, much easier to fix than an oral tube and is more readily tolerated.

Nasal intubation is preferred for long-term ventilation and is the route of choice in neonates and young children. Under the age of 2 years the larynx is narrower than the nasal passages.

Choice of tube

Plastic tubes are now widely used, and are much less irritant than red rubber tubes; a radio-opaque marker makes them visible on x-ray. In selecting the size of tube it is important to choose one that passes easily through the larynx, so minimizing trauma. In adults this is usually one with an internal diameter of 8–9 mm for men, and 7–8 mm for women. It is harder to give figures for children because the size of the larynx and trachea does not always relate to age. Sizes range from 3 mm in an infant to 5 mm in a child over 5 years of age.

For older children and adults, cuffed tubes are used. Inflating the cuff abolishes air leaks during ventilation and prevents aspiration around the tube. Uncuffed tubes are used in neonates and young children because of the small size of the trachea.

After intubation, the air entry to both lungs is checked; a tube inserted too far passes down the right main bronchus and the left lung is not ventilated. Once in a satisfactory position, it is fixed by material tape. The main complications that can arise at each stage of intubation are listed in Table 17.4.

Table 17.4 Complications of endotracheal intubation

During intubation	Damage to the larynx Intubation of the right main bronchus
whilst *in situ*	Obstruction: kinking secretions Displacement Pressure on the vocal cords Pressure on the trachea from the inflated cuff
After removal	Hoarseness Stridor Permanent laryngeal damage Tracheal stenosis

Damage to the larynx from pressure and movement of the tube is common. After short intervals this may only be superficial but after long periods, expecially if the tube has been inadequately fixed or is too large, deep ulceration of the larynx can occur. Healing of the more severe lesions causes fibrous scars, narrows the larynx and affects speech.

Damage to the trachea is caused by the pressure of the inflated cuff which interferes with the capillary circulation in the lining mucosa and a number of complications can develop (Table 17.4). Cuff pressure exerted on the tracheal wall should be as low as possible and it has been shown that high residual volume low pressure cuffs cause less damage than those with a small diameter and small residual volume. With the latter types the cuff becomes hard when inflated to the point of giving an adequate seal. The high residual volume cuffs are longer and are actively deflated for insertion (see Fig. 17.3). Intermittent deflation of the cuff does not confer any advantages.

The overall incidence of serious complications is around 5 per cent and, because of the effects on the larynx, if ventilation is required for more than ten days a tracheostomy should be performed. This spares the larynx, but the trachea is still exposed to pressure from the cuff of the tracheostomy tube.

Tracheostomy

Under most circumstances the operation is carried out under general anaesthesia. The neck must be fully extended and a short (5–7 cm) transverse incision is made mid-way between the cricoid cartilage and the suprasternal notch. The tracheal cartilages are exposed in the mid-line, dividing the isthmus of the thyroid gland if necessary, and the trachea is opened between the second and third rings. A window is then cut out by removing the second and third or third and fourth rings. Some surgeons fashion a flap by using a U-shaped incision. The lip of this flap is then stitched to the skin and forms a convenient guide into the trachea when the tracheostomy tube has to be changed. On completion of the operation the endotracheal tube is removed; a cuffed tracheostomy tube of the largest size that will fit comfortably is inserted and the cuff inflated (Fig. 17.4).

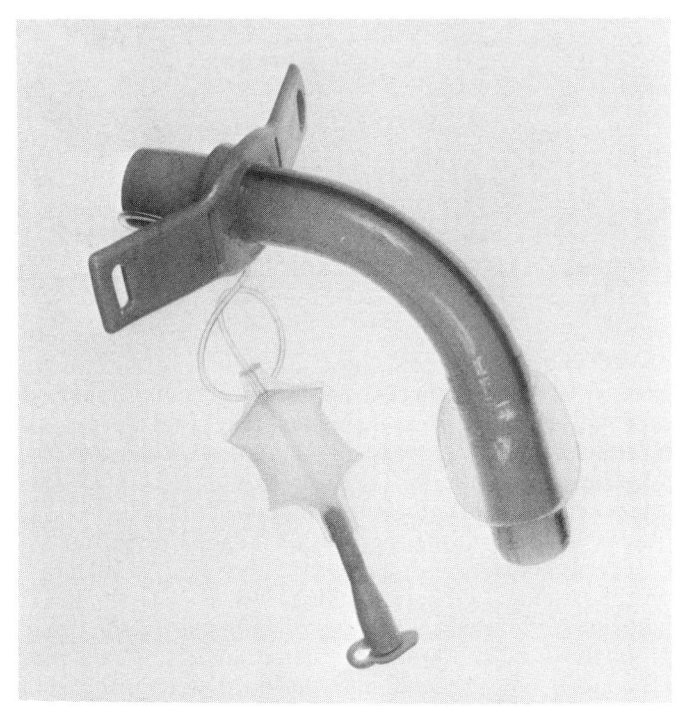

Fig. 17.4 Tracheostomy tube.

Starting IPPV

Typical starting values for an adult are tidal volume 12–15 ml/kg body weight, respiratory frequency 10–14 per minute and an inspiratory/expiratory ratio of 1:2. In hypoxaemic failure the inspired oxygen concentration is increased as required. The airway pressure that develops is determined by the size of the tidal volume, the compliance of the lungs, the resistance of the airways and the type of ventilator. Either a fall in compliance or an increase in airway obstruction will increase the pressure when a volume-cycled ventilator is being used. It is measured in centimetres of water (or kilopascals) and commonly lies between 15 and 40 cmH_2O (1.5 and 4.0 kPa) although in some instances pressures of 50–60 cmH_2O (5–6 kPa) may be required to maintain adequate ventilation.

After a period of ventilation with the initial settings, their adequacy is checked by measuring the arterial blood gases and any necessary adjustments are made.

In the early stages of ventilation, patients are often unable to adjust to the ventilator. They are restless, struggle and breathe out of phase; this reduces the efficiency of ventilation, increases the risk of displacing the tube and also the likelihood of damage to the larynx. It is therefore absolutely essential that the patient is rendered comfortable, quiet and co-operative. Except in the unconscious patient, this will require much explanation, reassurance and probably the use of sedatives and analgesics such as diazepam, papaveretum or phenoperidine. In the most severe cases the patient may have to be paralysed with a neuromuscular blocking drug, curare or pancuronium; when these are used the patient must always be fully sedated, for to be awake and paralysed is a terrifying experience.

It is also helpful, in this respect, initially to slightly hyperventilate the patient to reduce the natural drive to breathing. The rate of the ventilator should be sufficient to avoid the patient's having 'to wait' for the next breath. Large tidal volumes ensure that all areas of the lung are inflated. If the combination of tidal volume and frequency necessary for these purposes produces too high a minute volume, a mechanical 'dead-space' in the form of an extra length of ventilator tubing (15 cm each time) can be added to the circuit.

Benefits of IPPV

IPPV supports ventilation, improves ventilation/perfusion abnormalities by opening alveoli previously closed, and allows the inspired oxygen concentrations to be accurately controlled. Exhausted patients are able to rest and sedation can be given without fear of depressing natural respiration. The tracheal tube enables effective removal of any excess secretion.

Problems of IPPV

Mechanical problems stem from obstruction and displacement of the tracheal tube, and leaks or breaks in the ventilator circuit.

Circulatory disturbances. The increase in intrathoracic pressure produced by IPPV initially reduces venous return to the heart, cardiac output falls and the patient becomes hypotensive. This can be quite marked in patients with neurological disorders. The effect is usually short lived because physiological compensation occurs, producing a higher venous filling pressure to the heart. Patients on ventilators also have a tendency to retain water—which must be remembered when managing their fluid balance.

Infection Ventilators and humidifiers are potential sites of bacterial colonization and present hazards of auto- and crossinfection.

Oxygen toxicity. Oxygen in high concentrations (greater than 60 per cent) is toxic to the lungs. Concentrations in excess of this, including pure oxygen, can be given to an intubated patient but should be avoided if at all possible.

Pneumothorax. The positive airway pressure may rupture a weak part of the lung, causing a pneumothorax. This is always a serious complication and facilities for inserting a chest drain should be readily to hand.

Positive end-expiratory pressure (PEEP)

As the term 'positive end-expiratory pressure' implies, the fall of airway pressure during expiration is not allowed to reach the usual zero level but is held at some positive value (See Fig. 17.1). PEEP is usually applied in increments of 5 cmH_2O up to or occasionally above 15 cm. It increases the level of lung inflation at the end of expiration and so prevents the alveoli closing. This increases oxygen transfer by improving the ventilation/perfusion ratio. The rise in arterial P_{O_2} obtained by its use enables the oxygen concentration in the inspired air to be reduced. It should be introduced when conventional IPPV cannot support an arterial P_{O_2} of 60 mmHg (8 kPa) using an inspired oxygen concentration of 60 per cent. Because it increases further the intrathoracic pressure venous return to the heart is affected and cardiac output is reduced. Too high a level may diminish this to such an extent that, in spite of the increased arterial oxygen tension, the total oxygen supplied to the tissues (oxygen content of the blood × blood flow) is reduced. For each patient there is an optimum level of PEEP related to these considerations.

The higher airway pressures and increased lung distension also slightly increase the risks of pneumothorax, pneumomediastinum and subcutaneous emphysema—complications collectively referred to as 'barotrauma'.

A continuous positive airway pressure (CPAP) can also be applied to patients who are breathing spontaneously. This is of value in treating the respiratory distress syndrome of the newborn and sometimes in weaning patients from IPPV.

Other measures

When inspired oxygen concentrations in excess of 60 per cent together with high levels of PEEP fail to oxygenate the arterial blood adequately, the lung function, by inference, must be severely impaired. Not surprisingly, in such situations mortality is high; two additional measures, however, can still be tried.

1. *Hypothermia*. Lowering the patient's body temperature to 32°C reduces the oxygen requirements of the tissues and may increase the overall oxygen tension.
2. *Extracorporeal oxygenation* using a membrane oxygenator. This has had limited success in special centres but is associated with a number of serious complications, particularly haemorrhage. Also, in the cases that are severe enough to consider its use the lung disease may be irreversible.

Weaning from respiratory support

In general, once the respiratory failure has improved to a point where total ventilator support is judged to be unnecessary, weaning can be commenced. The complete process is divided into three phases:

1. weaning from the ventilator;
2. weaning from tracheal intubation;
3. weaning from additional oxygen.

It can range from a simple to an extremely complex and sometimes unpredictable process. Just as a number of factors contribute to the need for ventilation, there are several on which successful weaning depends.

After short periods of ventilation it may be possible to discontinue the support abruptly and completely; where it has been prolonged, however, weaning is more protracted and usually accomplished by gradually increasing, in a periodic manner, the length of time the patient is off the ventilator. During the periods of spontaneous ventilation, all other forms of respiratory care are continued and oxygen is given by a T piece attached to the tube. The patient may require some additional help from an assist or triggered ventilator. Intermittent mandatory ventilation (IMV) can be useful at the start of weaning. This technique makes it mandatory for the patient to breathe spontaneously whilst still on the ventilator and the machine delivers a 'breath' at pre-set intervals which can be progressively increased until the patient's ventilation is entirely spontaneous.

The whole weaning process requires careful and detailed supervision and can last from a few hours to several days, weeks or even months. Once the patient is able to breathe sufficiently well without support, the endotracheal tube can be removed.

Extubation

Extubation must be planned as carefully as intubation. After informing the patient, secretions are removed by suction from the mouth and trachea, the cuff is deflated and the tube removed during expiration. Any stridor that may follow extubation is usually short lived and in most instances responds to humidification. Occasionally, intravenous hydrocortisone may be needed. After removing the tube, oxygen therapy will then be gradually reduced over a period of time according to the value of the arterial P_{O_2}.

Antibiotics

Bacterial infections causing respiratory failure are treated with the appropriate antibiotics. Samples for bacteriology should always be taken before treatment is commenced. In severe infections they have to be started immediately before positive laboratory identification of the responsible organisms is available and, as in bacteriaemic shock, antibiotics with a wide range of activity are needed. A combination of penicillin, flucloxacillin and gentamicin is an excellent 'best guess' regimen for severe, unidentified pulmonary infections. It covers the possibility of pneumococcal, staphylococcal and a range of Gram-negative infections.

There is no evidence that the occasional practice of using antibiotics prophylactically reduces the risk of acquiring infection during ventilation. Indeed, the whole practice of unnecessary antibiotic therapy in ITU patients needs to be strongly condemned, for it has a number of very undesirable results. The patient can become colonized by resistant organisms which can produce severe invasive infections. *Pseudomonas* and *Proteus* species are common examples, along with various fungi. These will disappear once the broad spectrum antibiotics are discontinued.

Steroids

Except in severe asthma, there is little evidence that steroids have any value; however, they are often used in severe failure, particularly that associated with trauma or shock. Methylprednisolone (30 mg/kg) or dexamethasone (5 mg/kg) are currently the steroids of choice.

Acute-on-chronic respiratory failure

This is a problem quite different from that of acute respiratory failure. Patients with chronic respiratory failure often have considerable prior disability which cannot be improved by treating the acute exacerbation, and after each episode it is usually somewhat greater.

Treatment consists of controlled oxygen therapy, antibiotics and aggressive physiotherapy. In general, IPPV should be avoided in those patients with marked chronic disability because, once started, it may have to be continued for a very long period and weaning, if possible at all, may take an even longer time. CPAP is particularly helpful in weaning this group of patients.

In a small group of patients, respiratory stimulants such as doxapram or nikethamide might be of help, but on the whole they have little part to play in the treatment of respiratory failure and can induce unpleasant side-effects.

18

Equipment for respiratory care

Equipment for respiratory care forms a large part of the equipment in any ITU. It includes a wide and diverse number of items, ranging from sophisticated mechanical ventilators to common or garden plastic tubing. There are, however, three main categories: equipment for oxygen therapy, humidification of inspired gases and automatic ventilation.

Equipment for oxygen therapy

Oxygen is widely used for correcting the hypoxaemia of acute respiratory failure and for controlling the hypoxaemia of chronic respiratory failure. This distinction, between correcting and controlling, has to be appreciated because it has important therapeutic implications and has influenced the design of oxygen masks.

In general, patients with acute failure have normal respiratory control and can be given oxygen in any amount sufficient to fully correct the hypoxaemia. The situation is, however, different in chronic and acute-on-chronic failure where respiratory control is abnormal and a degree of hypoxaemia is a necessary stimulus for breathing. Too rapid correction will remove this drive; carbon dioxide then accumulates in the blood, the patient becomes drowsy and later comatose. In these patients, therefore, oxygen has to be given in gradually increasing concentrations.

There is no reason for any patient to be given more oxygen than is required; because it is so freely available from wall outlets there is a tendency to use it in a far too cavalier fashion. Like any drug, if given in excess it can, and does, produce serious side-effects.

Non-intubated patients

For the majority of non-intubated patients some form of facemask is used. The masks now available provide a wide range of oxygen concentrations, ranging from 24 per cent up to 60–70 per cent; as previously stressed, however, it is not possible for a patient to receive 100 per cent oxygen via a facemask.

In the past, it was customary to classify oxygen masks into controlled types, which provided relatively low but accurately measured concentrations, and uncontrolled varieties, which gave high concentrations but with less accuracy. This division has, however, become redundant because controlled oxygen therapy can now be provided at a concentration of 60 per cent whilst a number of previously 'uncontrolled' masks have been modified for accurate control. For this reason, in this chapter the various masks and devices for giving oxygen are not divided into such groups and are described individually.

Ventimasks (Fig. 18.1)
These were introduced in 1966 to provide a range of accurately controlled oxygen concentrations. Oxygen is delivered to the base of the mask through a nozzle with a fine hole. The gas passes through this at a high velocity and creates a turbulent flow in the wider ventitube, around which are several holes open to the atmosphere. The oxygen passes these and sucks in air by the Venturi effect; the air and oxygen are well mixed by the turbulence. The quantity of air entrained, and hence the final oxygen concentration, depends upon the size of the vent holes and the rate of oxygen flow.

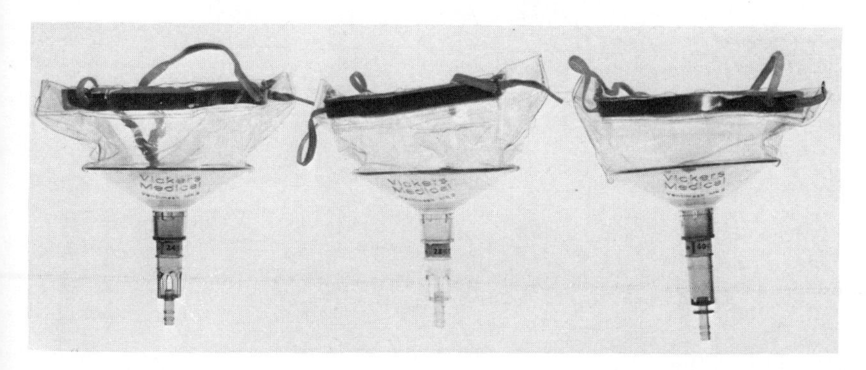

Fig. 18.1 Ventimasks.

The original Ventimasks have recently been modified to be smaller and lighter (Mk 2), and the range includes oxygen concentrations of 24, 28, 35, 40 and 60 per cent; the different masks each have an individual colour-coded Venturi. They are comfortable to wear, and the introduction of the 60 per cent mask enables accurate control at this high concentration. The Mk 2 range also includes a humidifier adaptor for wide-bore, light-weight tubing, essential for use with intubated patients.

Mixomasks
These are based on the same principle as the Ventimask and provide oxygen concentrations of 24, 28, 31, 35 and 40 per cent.

The Hudson mask (Fig. 18.2)
This is now widely used for administering high concentrations of oxygen. It is moulded in clear green plastic and, by varying the oxygen flow through it between 2 and 12 litres per minute, it gives concentrations from 23 to 76 per cent. (NB. The high figure is provided by the mask but not received by the patient.) A wide-bore gas entry point enables ventilator tubing to be attached. More recently, masks with variable vents have been marketed and different concentrations can be 'dialled'.

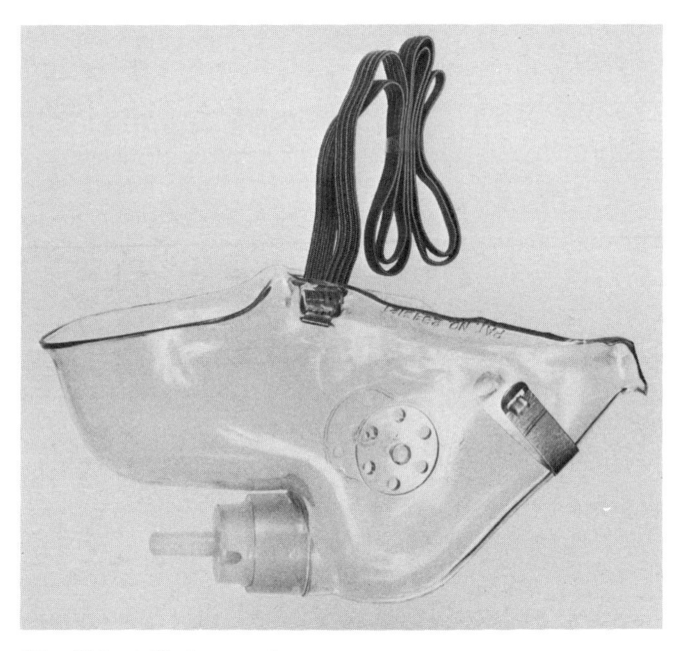

Fig. 18.2 A Hudson mask.

Nasal spectacles (Fig. 18.3)
These are useful in patients who cannot tolerate a facemask. Gas flow enters through two short prongs which are inserted into the nose. They have the advantage of not having to be removed during eating, drinking or physiotherapy, so avoiding wide fluctuations in inspired oxygen concentration. Accurate control of oxygen concentration is not possible and ranges from 25 to 40 per cent, with flow rates of 1–4 litres per minute. Mouth-breathing does not effect the concentration.

With all types of mask it is essential to ensure that the patient wears them properly all the time; intermittent oxygen therapy can have deleterious effects. This can be a difficult and frustrating task for the nurse because many of the patients are restless and confused.

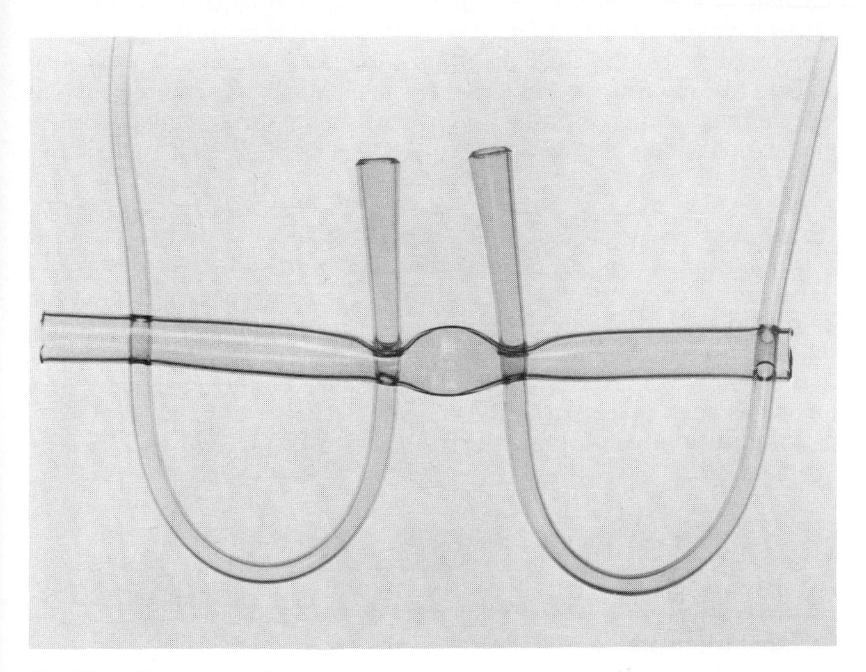

Fig. 18.3 Nasal spectacles.

Children and neonates

The restlessness of babies and young children and the unsuitable size of commercially available facemasks makes their efficient use impossible. Neonates and small infants are most easily nursed in an incubator into which oxygen can be introduced. Older children can be cared for in oxygen tents, but these are cumbersome to use and have to be disturbed to carry out essential nursing procedures. They also constitute a fire hazard because of the large enclosed volume of oxygen. Concentrations of 27–80 per cent can be achieved inside the tent.

Head-boxes are simple devices that fit loosely around the head and confine the oxygen-enriched atmosphere. They can also be used for applying CPAP.

Humidification is recommended when high concentrations of oxygen have to be given for more than one or two days.

Hyperbaric oxygen

Oxygen can be given at a pressure of more than 1 atmosphere if the patient is placed in a rigid chamber capable of withstanding pressures of 2, 3 or 4 atmospheres. Oxygen at such pressures increases the amount dissolved in the blood from 2 ml/100 ml (2 ml/dl) at 1 atmosphere to 8 ml at 4 atmospheres. The principle has been used to treat carbon monoxide poisoning and overwhelming anaerobic infections but is not widely available.

Intubated patients

If patients are being ventilated, the required concentration of oxygen is provided via the ventilator circuit. for intubated patients breathing spontaneously, necessary oxygen can be provided through a T piece connection attached to the endotracheal or tracheostomy tube or via a mask placed over the end of the tube.

In all intubated patients the inspired gases have to be artificially humidified.

Equipment for humidification

A humidifier has to provide gas to the trachea at a temperature of between 30 and 37°C and at a humidity of 34–44 mg H_2O/litre. It must be simple to use, easy to clean and sterilize, and electrically safe particularly from the point of view of over-heating. The factors affecting the efficiency of any humidifying device are:

1. The time of contact between the gas and the water.
2. The surface area involved in gas/water contact.
3. The temperature of the water.

The respiratory complications that arise when temperature and humidity are neglected are a direct consequence of drying of the tracheal mucosa. The sputum becomes tenacious and encrusted in the trachea, and atelectasis and secondary infection occur in the lungs.

Methods

Heat and moisture exchangers (artificial noses)
These devices are connected directly to the endotracheal tube or tracheostomy. They consist of rolled paper or metal mesh gauze. During expiration the warm wet gases pass through the network,

water condenses out and some heat is retained. In the next inspiration this heat and moisture is transferred to the incoming gases. The exchangers are not very efficient and have to be changed frequently. Their clinical use is very limited, being best suited to those tracheostomied patients with few secretions who are in the final stages of being weaned from humidification.

Nebulizers

Nebulizers produce microdroplets of water in the inspired gas.

In the gas-driven type, a jet of compressed gas entrains the water from a reservoir which may be heated. Nebulizers have serious disadvantages; there is heavy condensation in the delivery tubing and they are difficult to clean and sterilize. On balance, they are not a suitable type of humidification.

Mechanically activated nebulizers produce smaller droplets by dropping water, either onto a disc rotating at high speed or onto a crystal vibrating at high frequencies (ultrasonic). Very high levels of humidity can be achieved in this way, so much so that there is a risk of producing water intoxication. they pose a greater risk of infection because the smaller particles pass further into the lungs. The potential dangers of these humidifiers appear to outweigh the advantages of their high performance.

Cold water humidifiers

There are a number of types of cold water humidifiers where gas is either forced across or bubbled through water at room temperature. Their efficiency is not good enough for patients whose upper respiratory tract is bypassed.

Hot water humidifiers (Fig. 18.4)

With this type of humidifier gas is blown over, or bubbled through, heated water. The temperature of the water is regulated to achieve the optimum temperature in the airways. Over-heating is a particular danger and should be constantly looked for. Safety features to protect against this hazard are usually incorporated into the design.

At present, this form of humidifier is the most suitable and reliable for use in an ITU.

Ventilators (Fig. 18.5)

There are now in existence a plethora of different ventilators, varying not only in appearance but also in price. All, however, provide the same basic function: namely, that of moving respiration gases in and out of a patient's lungs and they are accordingly constructed of similar functional elements.

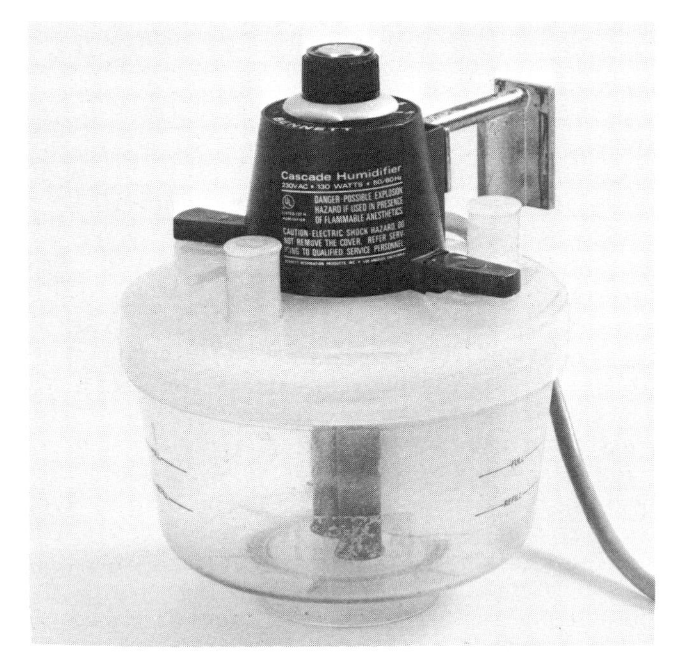

Fig. 18.4 A hot water humidifier.

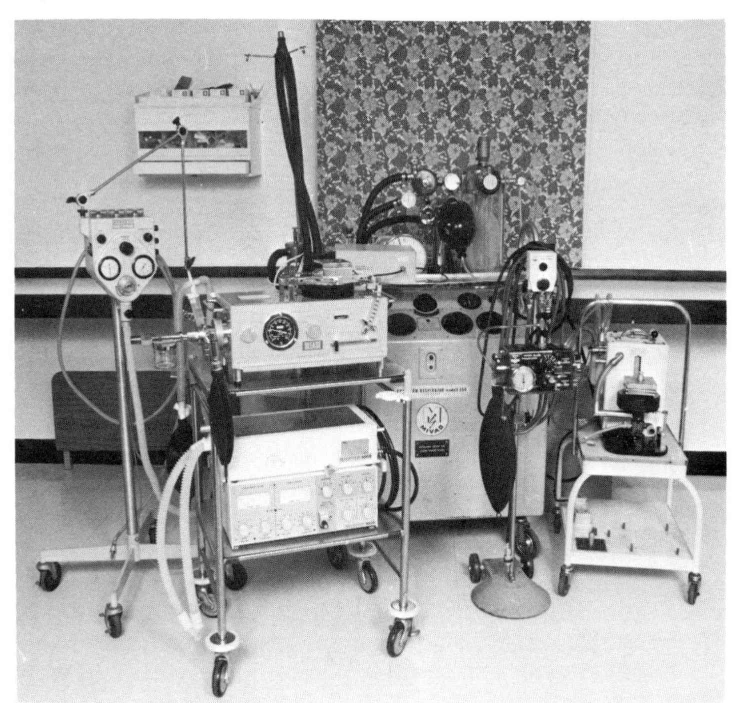

Fig. 18.5 A collection of ventilators.

Inflation of the lungs is achieved by supplying a positive pressure to the airways, and deflation by allowing time for the lung gases to expel the gases—the phases of inspiration and expiration. A ventilator therefore must have a means of changing (cycling) from one phase to the other, and a ventilator cycle is divided into four parts:

1. inspiration;
2. the cycle from inspiration to expiration;
3. expiration;
4. the cycle from expiration to inspiration.

With the flow of gases into the lungs during inspiration the pressure in the airways rises. The magnitude and pattern of this depends upon the size of the tidal volume, the flow rate of the inspiratory gases, the resistance of the airways and the compliance of the lungs, so that the overall pattern reflects the combined characteristics of the ventilator and the patient's lung.

At a certain point in the inflation, inspiration stops and expiration starts. The timing of this change may be determined by the volume of gas that has gone into the lungs (volume cycling), the level the pressure has risen to in the airways (pressure cycling), or a pre-set interval (time cycling). Expiration is a passive process affected by the recoil of the lungs and chest wall, during which the airway pressure falls back to zero. The time at which the next cycle starts depends on the rate of the ventilator. In some instances the ventilator cycles by sensing a negative pressure produced by the patient's own breath (patient cycling or triggering).

Classification

There are essentially two classes of ventilator: volume and pressure.

Volume generators

These deliver a pre-set tidal volume, and do so in spite of any changes in airway resistance or lung compliance. When inflation becomes more difficult, such a ventilator has sufficient reserve power to force the full volume of gas into the lungs, with a corresponding increase of airway pressure.

Cycling occurs after the set inflation has been completed (volume cycling) or after a fixed time interval (time cycling). In a purely time-cycling machine, if the inspiratory time is too short relative to the volume, then it will cycle before the full tidal volume has been achieved. It is therefore possible to have these two means of cycling linked to a ventilator in the functional class of a volume generator.

Pressure generators

These are designed to generate a pre-set airway pressure during inspiration, at which point they cycle to expiration (pressure cycling).

Should the airway resistance increase or compliance decrease, the set pressure will be attained with a smaller tidal volume and the minute volume will fall. The Bird series of ventilators are examples of pressure generators.

Alterations in lung characteristics during ventilation can therefore be detected in two ways: by changes in the inflation pressure using a *volume generator* and by changes in minute volume using a *pressure generator*.

Leaks in the ventilator circuit have more effect on the ventilation of the patient with volume generators, because the minute volume falls in proportion to the magnitude of the leak. A pressure generator, on the other hand, will continue inflation until the pre-set pressure is reached, so compensating for the leak unless it is very big, in which case the required pressure will never be reached.

In most forms of respiratory disease managed in an ITU, lung compliance and airway resistance may change frequently and over a wide range. During such fluctuations it is essential that the patient still receives the required minute ventilation, and for this reason a volume generator is preferred. In addition, it should have means for:

1. Controlling tidal volume, frequency and minute volume. Since these are interrelated, some ventilators provide independent control of tidal volume and frequency whilst in others minute and tidal volumes can be adjusted (minute volume dividers).
2. Accurately regulating the inspired oxygen concentration.
3. Adding a positive end-expiratory pressure. This can be obtained either by partially reducing the size of the expiratory orifice or by passing the expired gases through a spring-loaded or weighted valve or under a level of water.
4. Manual ventilation.
5. Controlling the ratio of inspiration to expiration. If fixed, this should be 1 : 2.
6. Easy cleaning and sterilizing.

Having fulfilled these six requirements, it should then be easy to use and understand, and be physically unobtrusive. Certain ventilators (usually the more expensive) have added facilities such as means of varying the inspiratory waveforms or adding an extra large tidal volume from time to time (sigh function). These inevitably add to the complexity of the machine and are, in many cases, of unproven value—examples of new technology outstripping clinical knowledge.

Paediatric ventilators

Most adult ventilators can be adjusted to give minute volumes down to around 2 litres but few are suitable for ventilating neonates. An ideal infant ventilator should have a widely adjustable rate (10–80 per minute), be able to generate high inflation pressures (up to 60 cmH_2O or 6 kPa) and small tidal volumes (10–60 ml).

19

Nursing care

The nursing care of patients in respiratory failure concerns both those patients who are breathing spontaneously and those who are being mechanically ventilated.

Non–ventilated patients

The specific aims of care are to:

1. Ensure that a clear airway is maintained.
2. Clear and remove secretions from the upper and lower respiratory tract.
3. Administer oxygen therapy effectively.

Maintaining a clear airway

Conscious patients, unless there are contraindications, should be nursed in a sitting position to help deep breathing and coughing. If the patient has to be nursed flat then the right and left lateral positions are used, with the head of the bed raised to an angle of 45° and the patient turned and re-positioned every two hours. Turning helps to prevent the development of pressure sores, deep vein thrombosis and joint stiffness. It also improves ventilation of the lung bases. Deeply unconscious patients require an artificial (Guedel) airway to prevent the tongue from falling back and obstructing the larynx. This is inserted with its tip directed towards the roof of the mouth, to avoid catching on the tongue and then rotated so that the tip comes to lie over the back of the tongue. If necessary, it can be fixed in position with adhesive strapping.

Clearing and removing secretions

Removing secretions from the upper and lower respiratory tract is vitally important to prevent obstruction of the air passages and the development of atelectasis. It is not always an easy task and problems can arise, particularly in patients with copious secretions and those who, for some reason, have difficulty in coughing. The problems are increased in confused, unco-operative or deeply unconscious patients.

The means that can be used to clear the airways include encouraging coughing and deep breathing, inhalations, postural drainage, nasotracheal suction and bronchoscopy. Such measures should be instituted early, when they are most likely to be beneficial.

Encouraging coughing and deep breathing

Proper coughing is probably the best method for preventing or treating atelectasis due to the retention of secretions. This must be done repeatedly. Pain and fear are common deterrents and patients need constant encouragement, explanation and reassurance. Postoperative patients with either thoracic or abdominal wounds usually find that coughing is easier when their incision is supported by firm pressure. In debilitated patients, compression of the chest during coughing is helpful.

Analgesics may be necessary but should not be given unnecessarily or in large doses because of the danger of depressing both the cough reflex and ventilation. Pre-mixed 50 per cent oxygen and 50 per cent nitrous oxide (Entonox) may prove helpful in this context; its effects wear off rapidly once it has been discontinued.

Inhalations

These can be of help in the conscious co-operative patient. Hot water with tincture of benzoin compound helps to loosen thick tenacious sputum but its administration must be carefully supervised because of the risk of the patient spilling the solution. A useful alternative, to prevent this hazard, is to use a disposable humidifier (Fig. 19.1) with the patient inhaling via a face mask. Inhalations of saline which help to liquefy secretions, or bronchodilators, can be given via a nebulizer.

Postural drainage

This moves secretions by gravity from the lungs into the trachea (Fig. 19.2) from where they can be removed by coughing or suction. It is chiefly the lung bases that require drainage. The manoeuvres should be timed to take place before the patient eats or is fed nasogastrically, in order to minimize the risk of aspiration.

Postural drainage is contraindicated in patients who are hypotensive, those with oesophageal reflux or severe head injury. It is not carried out during the 'running in' or 'running out' phase of

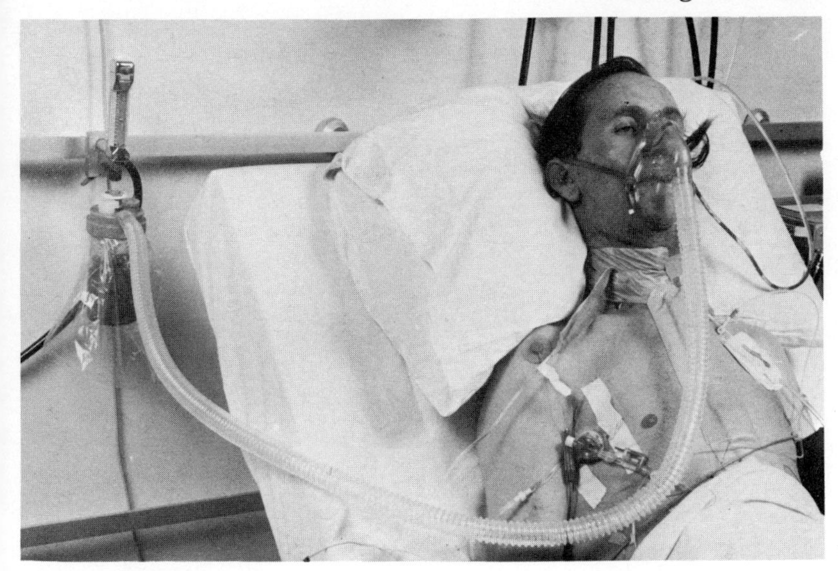

Fig. 19.1 A disposable humidifier being used for a tincture of benzoin compound inhalation. Lining the humidifier with a polythene bag prevents staining the container and enables it to be reused.

peritoneal dialysis and is better avoided after intracranial and cardiac surgery.

Nasotracheal suction

If coughing is ineffective, nasotracheal suction is used. This is an aseptic procedure, and, to reduce trauma, the catheter is lubricated with a gel. Conscious patients find it very uncomfortable and need reassurance. The catheter is passed through the nose into the pharynx and then, as the patient breathes in, it is rapidly but gently passed into the trachea. Suction is started, using an intermittent technique, as the catheter is slowly withdrawn.

The chief complication is damage to the lining of the respiratory tract, particularly the nasal passage, causing bleeding. It may also provoke a vasovagal reaction with bradycardia and hypotension. It is therefore contraindicated in patients with compound basal skull fractures, extensive fasciomaxillary injuries or coagulation disorders.

Bronchoscopy

If the measures outlined above fail, bronchoscopy with either a rigid or fibreoptic bronchoscope becomes necessary. Recurring accumulation of secretions can be removed, for a period, via an endotracheal tube left *in situ*.

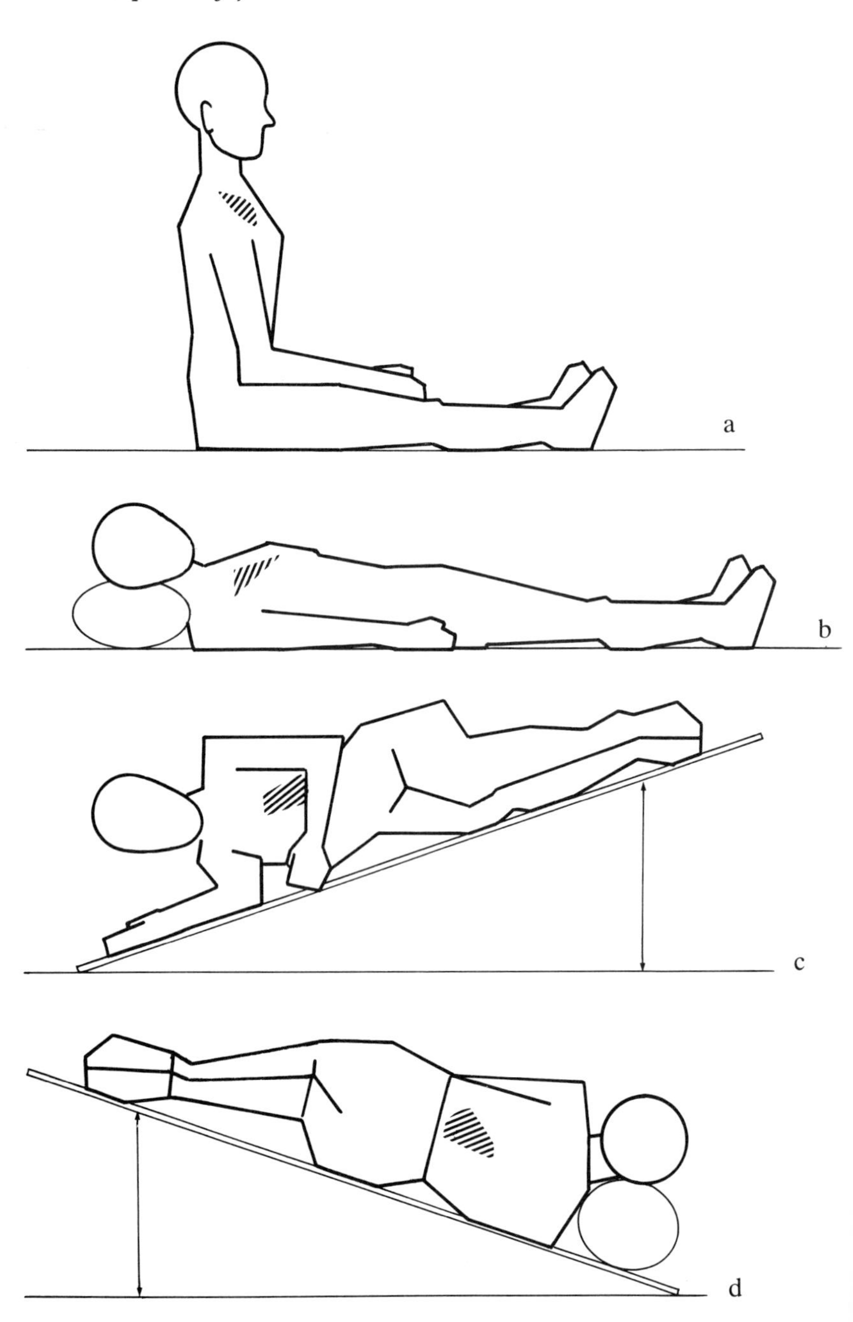

Fig. 19.2 The main positions for postural drainage. (a and b) Help secretions to drain from sections of the upper lobes. (c) From the left lower lobe. (d) From the left lower lobe.

Administration of oxygen

Face masks in general are uncomfortable but must be worn correctly at all times because of the dangers of intermittent oxygen therapy. This can be a particularly difficult task in confused and unco-operative patients.

Nasal spectacles are tolerated better and are easier to use when patients are restless and confused. Unlike face masks, they do not have to be removed for eating, drinking or mouth care and so provide uninterrupted oxygen therapy.

Whichever device is used, the nurse must repeatedly check its position and also the oxygen flow rate to it and the tubing connections.

Humidification

If oxygen has to be given for more than a few hours, it must be humidified in order to prevent drying and crusting of the secretions. A hot water humidifier is commonly used (Fig. 19.3) but must be checked regularly to ensure that:

1. Its container is not filled with water above the specified level and that the water level does not fall below the recommended 'refill' line.
2. The oxygen reaches the patient at a temperature near to 37°C. Because the gas cools as it passes along the tubing, the water in the

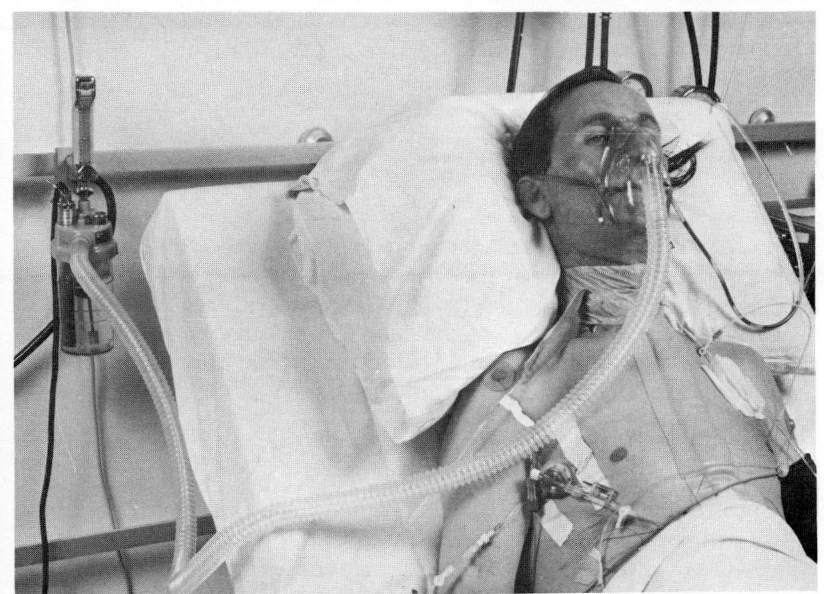

Fig. 19.3 A hot water humidifier.

humidifier needs to be heated to approximately 60°C. The temperature of the gas received by the patient can be accurately measured with a thermometer or crudely estimated by feeling the tubing (which should be comfortable to touch).

3. There are no leaks in the circuit.

With humidification, condensation and pooling of water occur in the tubing and must be drained away to prevent obstruction to the oxygen flow. The heat and moisture also cause deformity of the mask or spectacles and these need to be changed from time to time. Pressure from masks occurs on the bridge of the nose and tops of the ears, and these can be protected by inserting small pieces of gauze.

Hot water humidifiers are liable to become colonized by microorganisms, especially Gram-negative bacteria and, in particular, *Pseudomonas aeruginosa*. Bacterial contamination can be limited by keeping the water temperature at 60°C, which continuously pasteurizes the humidifier. The addition of an 0.02 per cent solution of chlorhexidine is an extra safeguard. The humidifier, tubing and oxygen mask or nasal spectacles must be changed daily.

Ventilated patients

The specific aims of care are to:

1. Ensure the position and patency of the endotracheal or tracheostomy tube.
2. Establish and maintain effective ventilation.
3. Clear and remove secretions.

Care of endotracheal tubes

Nasal

Nasal intubation is often preferred in conscious patients. The tube is more comfortable than one inserted orally, and may be so well tolerated that the patient is able to drink and eat soft foods.

Maintaining the patency of the tube can be difficult because of its narrow lumen, long length and tendency to kink. Bleeding from the intubated nostril is not uncommon, particularly after a difficult intubation.

Oral

The position of the oral tube may cause retching, coughing and nausea in conscious patients. Salivation is increased and stagnant collections of saliva in the mouth encourage bacterial growth. Special attention must be given to mouth care and excess saliva removed by suction.

Oral tubes are less likely to kink because they are shorter and wider than nasal tubes, although the patient may obstruct them by biting; an airway inserted into the mouth will prevent this. Maintaining patency is simpler because passage of a suction catheter is easier than via a nasal tube.

Securing the tube

Firm positioning is extremely important because the tube is the vital and most vulnerable link between the patient and the ventilator.

Inadequate fixation allows movement of the tube and so increases the likelihood of displacement. This is most likely to happen if the patient tries to cough or is moved. Movement of the tube may cause:

1. Damage to the tracheal mucosa, larynx and vocal cords.
2. Downward displacement into the right main bronchus with obstruction of the left main bronchus.
3. Upward displacement into the pharynx.

The nurse must be fully aware of the complications that can result from incorrect fixation. If at any time she is doubtful about the position of the tube, she must never attempt to move it without medical supervision.

Nasal tubes are readily secured with adhesive plaster (Fig. 19.4a), whilst material tape is used for oral tubes (Fig. 19.4b). The corners of the nostril or mouth respectively need to be protected from pressure by the insertion of small pieces of gauze or sponge material (Dalzaform). Continual changing of adhesive plaster makes the skin sore, so if for some reason frequent replacement is necessary material tape should be substituted. Material tape is changed daily and tied, with a reef knot, at the side of the face, never at the back of the neck where it might be confused with the tape of the patient's gown and accidentally untied.

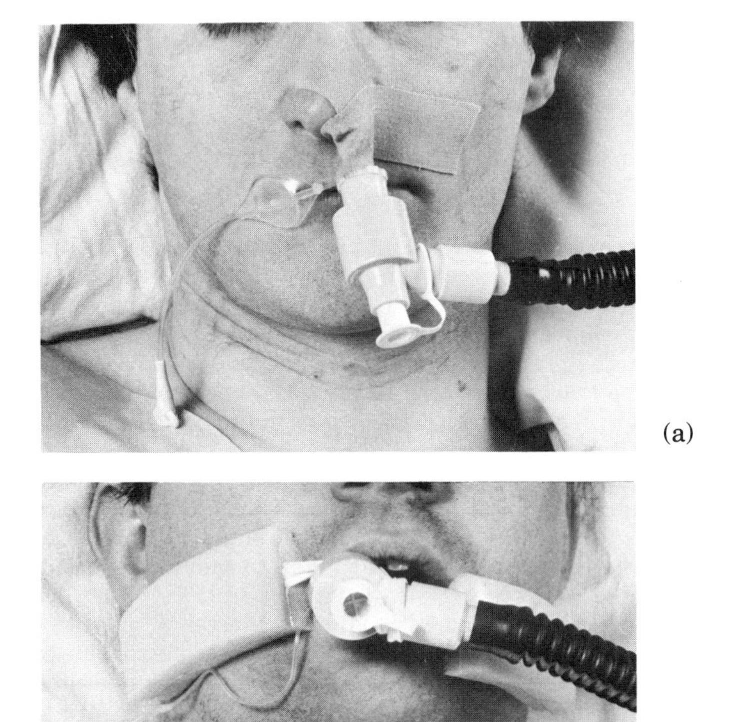

Fig. 19.4 (a) A nasal endotracheal tube secured in position with adhesive plaster.
(b) An oral endotracheal tube secured in position with material tape passed through sponge material to prevent pressure complications.

Care of tracheostomies

The stoma site

Initially the stoma site is observed for signs of swelling and bleeding. The limited presence of surgical emphysema is not a cause for concern. The tracheobronchial aspirate may at first contain a small amount of blood but this usually disappears within 24 hours.

The dressing is changed aseptically every four hours, or whenever excessively soiled by blood, exudate or secretions. This reduces the risk of bacterial contamination and promotes healing. The area is cleansed with normal saline, dried and a keyhole, non-adherent dressing is applied to prevent friction between the flanges of the tracheostomy tube and the skin. The frequency is decreased as the incision heals, and once healed the site is left exposed. If the stoma site is sutured, the stitches are removed on approximately the eighth day. A swab is taken each day from the stoma site for bacteriological culture.

The tracheostomy tube

Maintaining patency is not difficult because of its short length. The tube must be changed periodically, every fifth to seventh day, because its lumen becomes reduced by encrusted secretions.

The tube is secured in position by passing material tape through the flanges and tying its ends at the side of the neck, (for the same reason that material tape of an endotracheal tube is tied at the side of the face) (Fig. 19.5). It is important that the tracheostomy tube lies securely in position, for accidental decannulation can occur. Displacement into the right main bronchus is uncommon because of its short length, but continuous movement, especially in the region of the cuff, produces local oedema of the trachea and can result in ulceration, infection and erosion of the tracheal wall. Complete erosion can lead to a tracheo-oesophageal fistula.

Obstruction by secretions is uncommon if humidification is adequate and the tube is changed regularly. In the event of obstruction or accidental decannulation, prompt reinsertion of a new tube is necessary. Sterile tracheal dilators and a tracheostomy tube of the same size must therefore be kept at the bedside. Nurses must be given the opportunity whenever possible to learn how to change a tracheostomy tube.

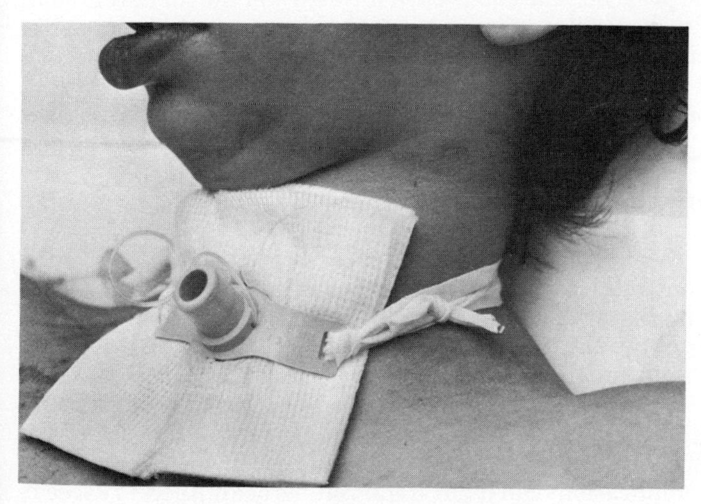

Fig. 19.5 A tracheostomy tube secured in position.

Changing a tracheostomy tube
When the tube is changed for the first time, it may be difficult because of the recent surgery and can result in slight bleeding, but after the initial change it is usually easier. To avoid discomfort, particularly for the apprehensive patient, a mild sedative beforehand is helpful. Oxygen or ventilation are discontinued only at the time of actual removal of the tube and are recommenced immediately the new tube is in place.

Changing a tracheostomy tube is a sterile procedure and requires two nurses—one to be the operator and the other the assistant. It is carried out as follows.

1. The procedure is explained to the patient.
2. The patient is placed either flat or in a sitting position with the neck extended.
3. The operator prepares the new tube, checking the integrity of the cuff and threading material tape through each flange. It is advisable to have a spare tube available, one size smaller than the existing tube, in case problems are encountered in inserting a tube of the same size.
4. The assistant unties the tapes of the tube in place.
5. The operator cleans around the stoma site. If the site is known to be infected, the assistant cleans the area using a separate dressings trolley and equipment.
6. The assistant sucks out secretions from the tube, then the mouth and finally the pharynx.
7. The assistant deflates the cuff and removes the existing tube.
8. The operator swiftly inserts the new tube, directing it through the stoma site, towards the posterior wall of the trachea and gently slides it into position. The cuff is then inflated and the tube secured in position. Tracheal dilators may be needed to widen the stoma site. Correct positioning of the tube is confirmed by observing the patient's colour and movements of the chest wall.
9. The patient is repositioned comfortably.

Cuff inflation

Inflation of the cuff of either an endotracheal or a tracheostomy tube is carried out once correct positioning has been confirmed. A re-breathing bag is attached to the tube, the lungs are inflated and movements of the chest observed. The cuff is then inflated with air, using a syringe, until an airtight seal is achieved. This is recognized by the disappearance of the distinctive 'hissing' sounds of escaping air from around the tube. A record should be kept of the size of the tube that has been inserted and the amount of air injected into the cuff. Cuff complications can occur if the volume of air injected exceeds the amount necessary to produce a seal (Fig. 19.6).

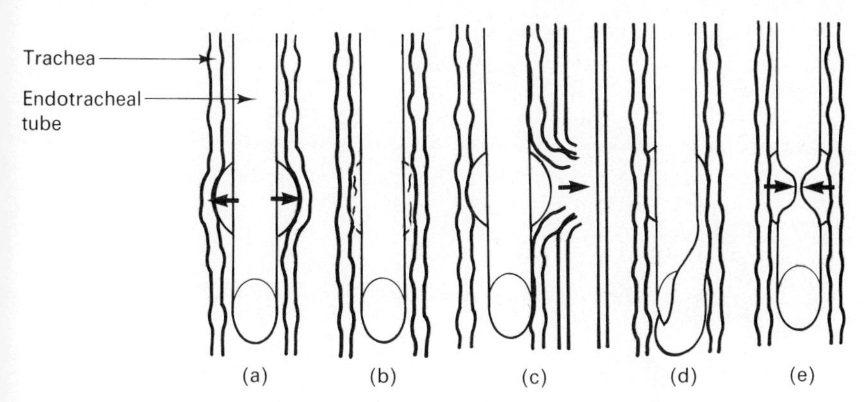

Fig.19.6 Complications that might result from over-inflation of the cuff. (a) Pressure on the tracheal wall. (b) Burst cuff. (c) Erosion of the tracheal wall. (d) Herniation. (e) Compression of the tube.

Establishing IPPV

All the equipment is sterilized and is prepared for use by checking that the:

1. Ventilator and humidifier are in working order.
2. Ventilator tubing is not damaged and is connected correctly.
3. Correct connections are available to attach the endotracheal or tracheostomy tube to the ventilator circuit.
4. Oxygen/air supply is connected to the ventilator and set to deliver the required flow rate.
5. Rate, volume and pressure settings on the ventilator are in accordance with instructions.
6. Ventilator alarm (if one is used) is working and that the alarm limits are set.

Suitable connectors are required to link the endotracheal or tracheostomy tube to the ventilator tubing. There has, in the past, been a confusing lack of standardization of such connectors and fittings, which meant having several different connectors available. Frequently a metal Magill or Nosworthy connector was used. These were heavy and may have been damaged or distorted by previous use and sterilization. As a result, the connection was weighty, often leaked and became disconnected from the ventilator tubing.

Apparatus is now manufactured with a standard 15-mm fitting or supplied with a 15 mm endotracheal tube adaptor. This is attached to a 15-mm swivel connector which is linked by a further 15-mm catheter mount adaptor to the catheter mount (Fig. 19.7). These connectors are all light weight and autoclavable and have overcome the disadvantages, in particular the danger of disconnection, of the other types.

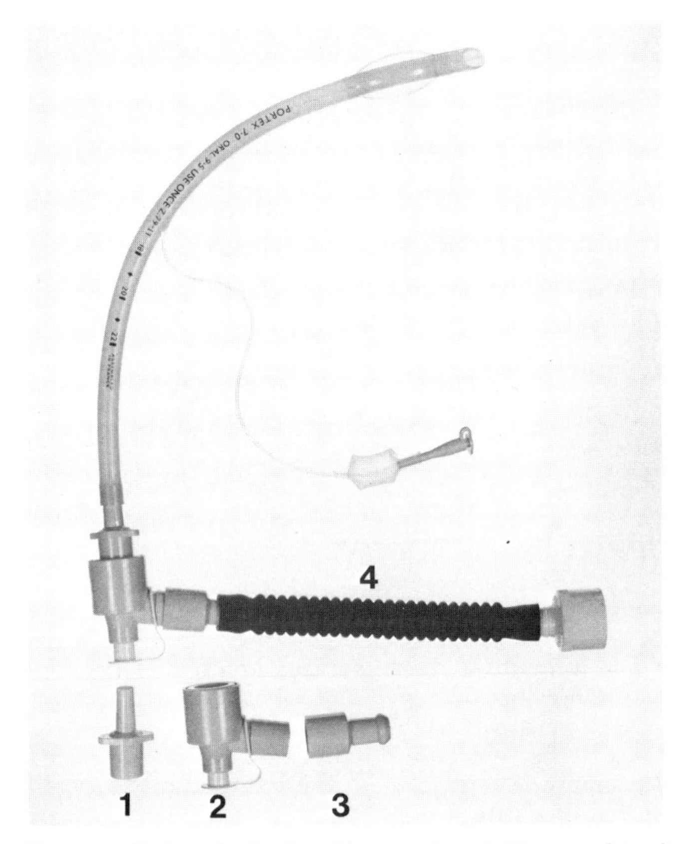

Fig. 19.7 Endotracheal tube with connectors: 1, 15-mm endotracheal tube adaptor; 2, swivel connector which can be moved in any direction; 3, 15-mm catheter mount adaptor; 4, catheter mount.

Maintaining IPPV

The effects of ventilation are assessed by observing the patient's colour and chest movements, and by recording the blood pressure and pulse rate. The first signs of ventilatory inadequacy and hypoxia may be tachycardia and hypertension. In addition, ventilatory measurements are recorded: these include the expired minute and tidal volumes, airway pressure and rate of ventilation (Fig. 19.8).

VENTILATOR O_2 FLOW l/min				4	4	4/3	3/2	2	2	2	2	2	2	2	2	2	2	2	2	2
AIR FLOW l/min				4	4	4/5	5/6	6	6	6	6	5	5	4	4	4	4	4	4	4
MINUTE VOLUME l/min					8·1	8	10	10	9	10·2	8·8	7·4	8·9	7·9	7·9	7·3	7·3	7·4	7·4	7·9
RATE/min				16	13	15	16	15	13	15	14	13	13	12	11	10	10	10	10	10
TIDAL VOLUME ml				600	620	610	710	700	610	690	575	600	610	640	640	630	650	640	650	635
INFLOW PRESSURE cm water					0/23	0/22	0/22	0/36	0/30	0/32	0/24	0/24	0/24	0/22	0/20	0/21	0/20	0/20	0/20	0/20
INSPIRE O_2 CONCEN %																				
HUMIDIFIER TEMP °C				6·5	6·5	6·5	7	7	7	7	6·5	6·5	6·5	6·5	6·5	6·5	6·5	6·5	6·5	6·5

Fig. 19.8 Ventilator observations.

Changes in these recordings can arise for a number of reasons and, because ventilatory volume, airway pressure and rate of ventilation are all inter-related, a single fault may produce changes in all of them. However, each one needs to be considered separately in the first instance. Fault finding must be carried out in a systematic manner, starting at the endotracheal or tracheostomy tube and ending at the gas supply (Fig. 19.9, p. 224).

Ventilatory observations

Expired minute and tidal volumes
These are measured by a respirometer, and many ventilators have one included. Condensation within the respirometer from the expired air can interfere with its accuracy and these ventilators have a means of bypassing the air flow between recordings.

A single recording of tidal volume may not be truly representative and the mean value of three should be taken; alternatively, the expired minute volume can be measured and divided by the rate of ventilation.

A decrease in minute volume occurs when the ventilator circuit leaks or is obstructed. With a volume-cycled ventilator, significant leaks lead to a fall in ventilation, whereas a pressure-cycled machine compensates for small leaks. The leak or obstruction is traced by checking the patency of the endotracheal or tracheostomy tube, cuff seal, connections, tubing (for kinking or pooling of water) and gas flow meter and its connections.

An increase in minute volume is less common and less serious. The reason is either an increase in the gas supply to the ventilator or the patient breathing between the ventilator 'breaths'. It is easily remedied by reducing the gas supply or, when clinically necessary, sedating the patient.

Airway pressure values are displayed on the ventilator, showing a peak on inspiration and a fall during expiration. Oscillation of the gauge needle between cycles signifies a patient breathing spontaneously.

A decrease in peak airway pressure is caused by a leak in the ventilatory circuit and, with volume-cycling ventilators, is associated with a decrease in ventilating volume. If there are no leaks, a fall in airway pressure probably represents an improvement in the patient's lung compliance.

An increase in peak airway pressure results from obstruction to the gas flow. It will not occur with pressure-cycled machines since they cycle once the pre-set pressure has been attained. It does, however, produce a fall in minute volume.

The obstruction is commonly in the endotracheal or tracheostomy

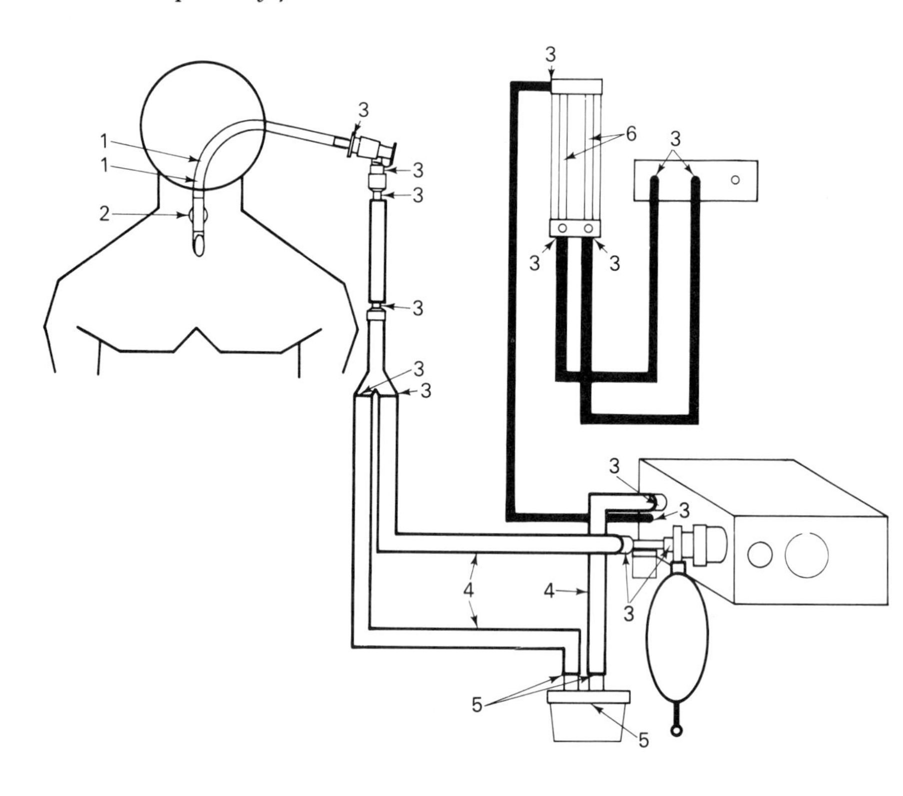

Fig. 19.9 Possible faults and their consequences.

	Fault	Consequence
1. *Endotracheal tube*	Secretions	Obstruction to the gas flow
	Kinked tube	Obstruction to the gas flow
1. *Tracheostomy tube*	Secretions	Obstruction to the gas flow
2. *Cuff*	Underinflated	Gas leakage
	Burst cuff	Gas leakage
3. *Connections*	Loose	Gas leakage
	Disconnection	Gas leakage/ventilation stopped
4. *Circuit tubing*	Pooling of water	Obstruciton to the gas flow
	Kinked tubing	Obstruction to the gas flow
	Damaged tubing	Gas leakage
5. *Humidifier*	Loose connections	Gas leakage
	Leakage around base and lid	Gas leakage
6. *Gas flow meter*	Increase in gas supply	Increase in inspired gases
	Decrease in gas supply	Decrease in inspired gases

tube due to secretions, kinking or the patient biting an oral tube or, in the ventilator tubing, due to pooling of water or kinking.

The ventilator rate may be displayed on the ventilator, but otherwise it will have to be counted.

Changes in the ventilator rate rarely occur in isolation. Usually they are associated with leaks or obstructions in the circuit.

In the presence of a possible ventilator fault, the nurse must always first check the clinical state of the patient. If this is satisfactory, then detection of the fault can proceed. When the patient is showing signs of insufficient ventilation, the nurse must start hand ventilation whilst waiting for assistance.

Humidification

The majority of ITU ventilators are used in conjunction with a hot water humidifier, a few with nebulizers.

Hot water humidifiers

These consist of a bath and a thermostatically controlled heating element which heats the water to a temperature of 55–60°C. The gases cool as they pass from the humidifier along the inspiratory tubing and reach the patient at a temperature of approximately 37°C.

To ensure the efficient and safe operation of the humidifier the checks mentioned previously are required. A thermometer can be used to record the water temperature but it is more appropriate to measure the gas temperature at the patient end of the delivery tubing. The greatest danger of a hot water humidifier is failure of the thermostatic control with over-heating of the water, the inspired gas temperature increases and may cause scalding of the trachea and lungs.

The humidity in the inspired gas causes water to collect in the ventilator tubing, particularly the dependent loops. For this reason the tubing should never be supported above the patient's head because of the obvious danger of water entering the lungs. The water must be removed from time to time to prevent obstruction to the gas flow. Many ventilators have a 'condensation trap' in the expiratory limb, but not all the moisture from the inspiratory or expiratory tubing collects in this. Excess water in the tubing has to be drained. In the inspiratory limb it may be drained back into the humidifier, or the tubing disconnected from the humidifier and drained into a receptacle. If the tubing is disconnected, speed is essential since the patient is not being ventilated during this period.

Bacterial contamination of a humidifier is serious because the bacteria are directed into the lungs. Preventive measures have already been described.

Nebulizers
Nebulizers require careful attention to ensure that the stipulated number of drops of water per minute does not increase or decrease. An adult usually requires eight to ten drops per minute. A fall in drop rate causes inadequate humidification, whereas an increase particularly in infants, may produce fluid overload.

Bacterial contamination is a risk with nebulizers; the equipment must be checked daily and only sterile water used.

General nursing care

A patient who is receiving artificial ventilation needs a nurse to be constantly present. The nurse must understand how the ventilator operates and be capable of hand ventilating the patient (rebreathing apparatus must be kept at the bedside). Regular observations are recorded on ventilation, the vital signs and fluid balance. All procedures likely to disturb the patient must be fully explained before they are carried out. The conscious patient will need repeated reassurance about his treatment and progress and that his inability to speak is only temporary.

When a patient is uncomfortable on a ventilator, breathing occurs out of sequence and the patient is restless, perhaps perspiring, flushed or cyanosed. Inflation pressures are variable with high or even negative values. The expired minute volume increases because of the patient's spontaneous breaths. This state is often referred to as 'fighting the ventilator' and should be corrected because it imposes additional stresses on the patient and interferes with optimal ventilation. If it is allowed to persist, it produces a vicious circle with the patient becoming more and more agitated and inadequately ventilated. The nurse must establish the cause of the problem by checking the whole of the ventilator circuit from the endotracheal or tracheostomy tube to the flow meter. If no fault can be found, it is justifiable to give the patient sedation.

Clearing and removing secretions

The presence of an endotracheal or tracheostomy tube prevents coughing and the removal of secretions is wholly dependent on tracheal suction. The frequency with which this needs to be carried out is dictated by the patient's pulmonary state.

Tracheal suction
A suction catheter is passed through the endotracheal or tracheostomy tube down to the carina. Straight, disposable, plastic catheters are widely used, and those with an open end and side holes are

thought to cause less trauma to the tracheal mucosa than do ones with a single side hole. The size of the catheter should be somewhat less than half the diameter of the endotracheal or tracheostomy tube. With larger diameter catheters there is a risk of too much negative pressure being applied to the lungs. Suction tubing and catheters should both be transparent so that the nature of the aspirate can be observed.

The vacuum pressure required to remove secretions is between 150 and 200 cmH_2O (15 and 20 kPa). Higher pressures will collapse the sides of the catheter and cause damage to the tracheal mucosa.

Tracheal suction is an aseptic procedure. A mask is worn by the operator and disposable gloves are used for handling the catheter. A new sterile catheter and glove are used for each aspiration. With the catheter held in readiness in the gloved hand, the nurse releases the connection to the endotracheal or tracheostomy tube with the other hand, and the catheter is passed down the tube to the carina. Suction is not applied until the catheter has reached the carina; the catheter is then withdrawn, using an intermittent technique which helps to reduce the amount of oxygen drawn into the suction apparatus. Rotation of the catheter is avoided because this causes tracheal invagination. When secretions are tenacious, instilling (with a syringe) 1–2 ml of normal saline down the endotracheal or tracheostomy tube helps to liquefy them and makes their removal easier.

Intermittent suction is achieved by inserting a Y connection between the suction tubing and the catheter. Suction is applied by occluding the limb of the Y. Alternatively, the catheter can be kinked at its proximal end or a catheter with a proximal finger hole used (Fig. 19.10).

Suction should not be applied for more than 15 seconds at a time without allowing the ventilator to provide two or three breaths. If prolonged, the patient may become hypoxic and bradycardic.

Physiotherapy

Not all secretions are responsive to suction alone. Physiotherapy is required to dislodge and move them from the small airways into the large ones so that they can then be removed by suction. There are two main techniques: bag-squeezing and postural drainage.

Bag-squeezing hyperinflates the lungs and mimics normal sighing and yawning. It expands the alveoli and prevents atelectasis by dislodging secretions. Squeezing must not be too vigorous because of the risk of producing a pneumothorax.

It is carried out using the manual bag on the ventilator circuit, an Ambu bag or a Waters' canister. Use of the bag on the ventilator circuit is a good method for teaching because the inflation pressure can be seen on the ventilator. The patient is placed flat in the lateral position and the rebreathing bag is connected to the catheter mount or the manual bag on the ventilator is operated. The oxygen flow rate is set at 15 litres and the lungs are rhythmically hyperinflated by

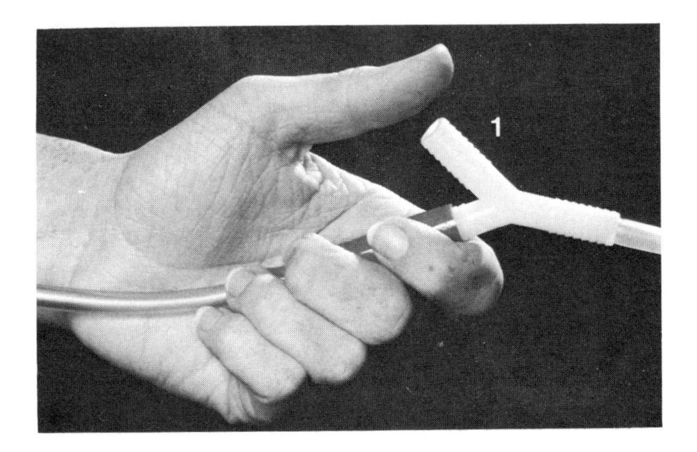

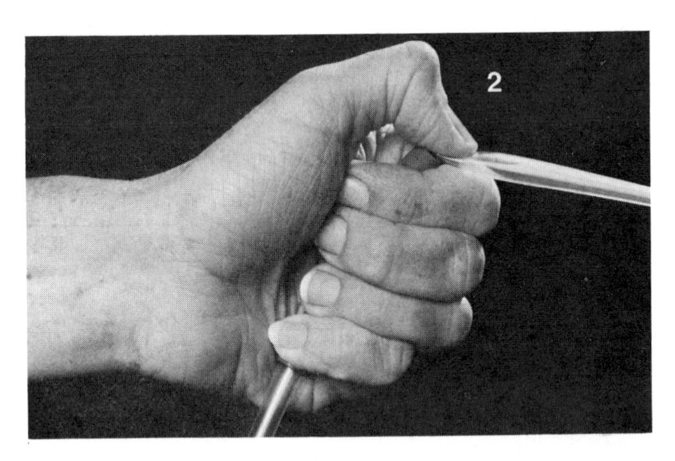

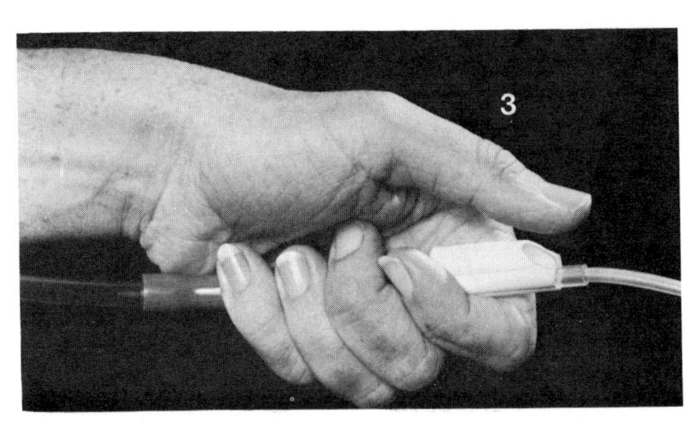

Fig. 19.10 Methods of intermittent suction: 1, using a Y connection; 2, kinking the catheter; 3, using a catheter with a proximal finger hole.

squeezing the bag. Several 'breaths' are necessary to dislodge secretions. When one lung has been treated, the patient is turned to the opposite side and the procedure is repeated. It should be carried out two-hourly where possible, but is contraindicated in patients who require uninterrupted IPPV (for example, patients with a flail chest) or those dependent on a high level of positive end expiratory pressure (PEEP).

Postural drainage, as previously described, moves secretions by gravity (see Fig. 19.2) and is used to encourage drainage of secretions in conjunction with bag-squeezing.

Weaning from ventilation

With adequate recovery of respiratory function, weaning can be commenced. The ease with which this is achieved is very variable. In patients who have been ventilated for a short time, it is nearly always possible for them to breathe successfully on their own straight away, whereas patients who have had long-term support will require progressive periods on and off the ventilator.

Methods of weaning

The various methods of weaning fall into two groups: continued support with gradual increasing periods of spontaneous breathing or, progressively diminishing support using either triggered ventilation or intermittent mandatory ventilation. One method may be more appropriate to a particular patient than another and often the most suitable method is found by trial and error. Whichever method is chosen, the principles must be explained to the patient with the assurance that this is a progressive step in his treatment. To begin with, the patient will need encouragement and reassurance until he regains confidence in his own ability to breathe.

Spontaneous breathing is carried out, sedation having been withheld for four hours, with a T piece attached to the endotracheal or tracheostomy tube through which humidified oxygen is supplied to the patient. When tracheal suction is required, the secretions are removed through the aspriation hole (Fig. 19.11) to ensure that the patient still receives some oxygen.

During the initial periods of spontaneous breathing the patient's pulse rate, respiratory rate and minute and tidal volumes are recorded every five minutes and the blood pressure measured every 15 minutes. The frequency of these observations is decreased once the patient shows signs of maintaining his own breathing. The nurse must encourage the patient to breathe deeply and watch for signs that indicate respiratory distress and hypoxia—tachycardia, tachypnoea, cyanosis and hypotension. No patient must be allowed to become frightened or exhausted. This can create a feeling of total dependence on the ventilator, resulting in doubt and apprehension about the next period of selfventilation.

The use of triggered ventilation and intermittent mandatory ventilation ensures that the patient receives a basic minute volume whilst making some respiratory effort.

Triggered ventilation requires the patient to make an effort to breathe. Initially the controls are adjusted so that only a slight respiratory effort from the patient provokes the delivery of the preset tidal volume. This is progressively changed, making the patient work harder until he breathes entirely on his own.

Intermittent mandatory ventilation provides a method by which the patient breathes spontaneously from an additional source of oxygen and air connected into the ventilator circuit, with the ventilator delivering 'breaths' at a pre-set rate. The rate at which the ventilator is set is gradually reduced as the patient becomes capable of taking over his own breathing. The effectiveness of the patient's breathing is assessed by the minute and tidal volumes.

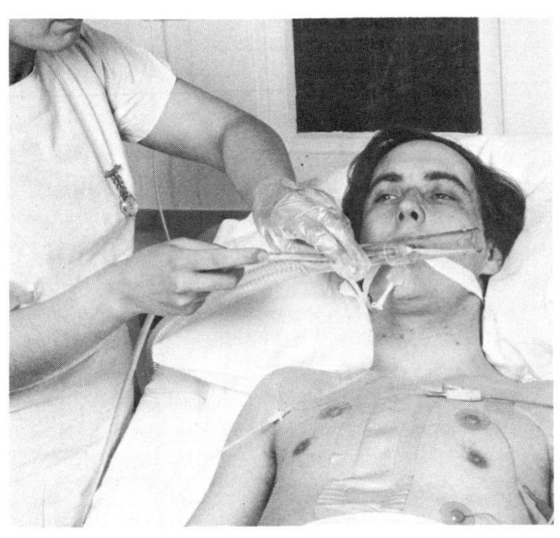

Fig. 19.11 T piece attached to an endotracheal tube. Secretions are being moved via the aspiration hole.

Removal of the endotracheal tube

Once normal respiration is established, the patient can be extubated. All the necessary equipment for re-intubation must be available. Tracheal suction is carried out and excess saliva sucked from the mouth.

The cuff of the tube is deflated and the securing tapes or adhesive plaster removed. A suction catheter is passed into the tube and suction, using the intermittent technique, is performed as the tube is withdrawn. After removal, the patient is asked to breathe deeply through the mouth, to exclude the presence of laryngeal stridor. Mild stridor can be effectively treated with steam inhalations.

Closing the tracheostomy

The tracheostomy tube is removed two to three days after completion of weaning. During this time the cuff of the tube is left deflated and checks made of the airway protective reflexes. This is usually done by simply noting the absence of coughing during eating and drinking. If doubt exists, the patient is given a small amount of coloured fluid to drink and then the tracheal contents are aspirated and inspected.

Prior to extubation the platic cuffed tube is often replaced by a silver one for at least a few days. Silver tubes have an inner tube and this needs to be removed and cleaned every two to four hours. It is soaked in sodium bicarbonate, cleaned with a small brush to remove secretions and sterilized before re-insertion.

On removal of the plastic or silver tube, an airtight dressing is applied (a firm pad of gauze strapped in position). The patient is instructed to apply pressure, with his fingers, to the stoma for talking and coughing. At first coughing may be relatively ineffective because of the air leak through the tracheostomy tract and suctioning may be necessary. Each time the dressing is soiled it is changed aseptically, the objectives being to prevent bacterial contamination of the stoma site and to keep it dry to promote healing. The stoma usually closes within five to ten days.

Section E

Renal and metabolic failure

20
Acute renal failure

Acute renal failure stems from a rapid deterioration in renal function and is characterized by a fall in glomerular filtration rate (GFR), oliguria and an accumulation in the body of water and those substances that are normally excreted in the urine. In the ITU the first manifestation is usually oliguria—a urine volume of less than 30 ml per hour. This dominates the early stages of diagnosis and treatment.

Classification

It is of great practical help to classify acute renal failure into three categories according to its cause: pre-renal, renal and post-renal.

Pre-renal failure is the result of a reduced cardiac output in hypovolaemic, cardiogenic or bacteraemic shock. The low cardiac output reduces renal blood flow and GFR; the oliguria is a direct consequence of the low GFR and a continuing response of the renal tubules to the action of ADH. In essence there is a state of reduced renal perfusion but intact function. The changes at this stage are reversible if the circulatory disturbance is corrected. If, however, treatment is delayed or ineffective, they progress and renal failure becomes established.

Renal failure follows, as described, from the pre-renal state when this has been severe or prolonged. In this context it is often referred to as 'acute tubular necrosis' or 'established renal failure'. 'Tubular necrosis' is a somewhat misleading term, for relatively little structural damage is apparent in the kidneys despite their marked impairment of function, and the latter description is preferred. It is usually a self-limiting condition, lasting a few days or weeks, and recovery from it is heralded by a diuresis.

In addition to renal ischaemia there are other factors which predispose to, or aggravate, the severity of the renal impairment. Susceptibility is increased during pregnancy and in association with jaundice (the hepatorenal syndrome). Certain drugs—for example, the aminoglycoside antibiotics—are nephrotoxic. Disseminated intravascular coagulation or the presence of increased quantities of circulating myoglobin (from muscle injury) or haemoglobin (from intravascular haemolysis) intensify any renal ischaemia.

Acute glomerulonephritis or acute pyelonephritis can cause renal failure without any preceding renal ischaemia.

Post-renal failure results from obstruction of the urinary tract by stones, tumours or blood clots. It may present with anuria rather than oliguria.

Biochemical disturbances

Nitrogen retention is a universal feature. The blood urea rises rapidly, especially in hypercatabolic patients, and the blood creatinine increases in proportion to the severity of the renal failure.

Hyponatraemia is common and usually signifies water overload.

Hyperkalaemia occurs primarily because of the reduced renal excretion of potassium but this is aggravated by an increased release from the cells in hypercatabolic states. It may rapidly reach life-threatening levels.

Metabolic acidosis is caused by a reduced excretion of hydrogen ions and the accumulation of the acid products of protein breakdown in the blood. Plasma bicarbonate and pH fall.

Clinical features

Oliguria is the presenting feature and its onset can be quickly recognized if the patient is already catheterized and urine volumes are being recorded hourly. Most of the other manifestations are secondary to fluid and electrolyte disturbances affecting other systems.

Respiratory. Dyspnoea is related to pulmonary oedema and metabolic acidosis.

Cardiovascular. Oedema and hypertension are a consequence of fluid overload; pericarditis is uncommon.

Gastrointestinal. Anorexia, nausea and vomiting are all common and are probably related to water overload. In some patients hiccoughs are troublesome and gastrointestinal bleeding may occur in advanced renal failure.

Neurological. Drowsiness, confusion, muscle twitching and coma are later manifestations and point to widespread metabolic disturbances.

Diagnosis

The diagnostic problem centres on the cause of the oliguria. The cause may be obvious, but mistakes will be made unless all possibilities are considered. Always start by ensuring that the urinary catheter is patent; blocked catheters still feature as a cause of oliguria or anuria.

Any possibility of a post-renal cause needs to be eliminated. If there is any likelihood of this, a straight x-ray of the abdomen followed by a high dose IVP should be carried out. An abdominal x-ray is always helpful to measure the size of the kidneys. If they are smaller than normal, some element of chronic renal failure may exist.

After exclusion of any possible post-renal cause, the differential diagnosis is then between pre-renal and renal causes which, in functional terms, is the difference between a reversible and an established condition. Observing the response to treatment is the only realistic way to resolve this problem.

If, as the low cardiac output is increased, the urine volume also increases, then clearly the condition is reversible. Should, however, the oliguria persist, established renal failure is likely to have developed. Analysis of the urine is helpful at this stage because if the kidneys are still capable of function, the urine will have a high specific gravity (greater than 1.020) and a high osmolality (greater than 400 mmol/kg).

Oliguria persisting in spite of an improved circulation is an indication to use diuretics, either frusemide in a high dose (1 g over four hours) or mannitol (200 ml of a 20 per cent solution). If they are ineffective, there is little point in giving further doses. Large doses of frusemide are ototoxic and mannitol can lead to circulatory overload and a hyperosmolar state.

No response at this stage signifies that the renal failure is established and a strict conservative regimen of treatment must be started.

Conservative management of established renal failure

The aim of conservative management is to keep the volume and composition of the body fluids as near normal as possible, in particular to prevent fluid overload, hyperkalaemia and acidosis. The regimen is as follows.

1. *Water intake is restricted* to 400 ml per day, to replace insensible loss, plus additional quantities equal to the urine volume and any other losses that may be present; sodium intake is also curtailed and

only overt losses are replaced. Weighing the patient daily gives an accurate guide to the state of fluid balance in this situation.

2. *A high calorie intake* of at least 2000 calories to minimize endogenous protein breakdown. This can be provided orally with carbohydrate solutions such as Caloreen or Hycal, but these may cause diarrhoea and cannot be used if the patient is vomiting. Intramuscular chlorpromazine or perphenazine will help to stop vomiting but sometimes it will only respond to dialysis. In hypercatabolic states more than 2000 calories are needed and must be provided with 50 per cent dextrose plus insulin or by fat solutions, intravenously. Protein intake is stopped initially but limited amounts may be necessary in the later stages to achieve a positive nitrogen balance. Anabolic steroids are sometimes given to reduce the rate of catabolism but their value is limited.

3. *Control of hyperkalaemia*, which is the most dangerous complication. No additional potassium must be given. Acute elevation of the serum potassium can be controlled for a limited period with the use of glucose and insulin and ion-exchange resins (Resonium-A).

4. *Correction of the metabolic acidosis*, when severe, by sodium bicarbonate; this treatment suffers, however, from all the disadvantages and limitations described in relation to its use in cardiac arrest.

5. *Treatment of any infections*, which are not uncommon complications and will increase the rate of catabolism. The urinary catheter should be removed to prevent the risk of a urinary tract infection. Prophylactic antibiotics are not indicated.

6. *Adjustment of drug therapy*: nephrotoxic drugs (Table 20.1) are avoided and the dose is adjusted of all drugs (including digitalis) that are eliminated via the kidneys.

Table 20.1 Some nephrotoxic drugs

Antibiotics	Other drugs
Gentamicin	Phenindione
Tobramycin	Phenacetin
Amikacin	Dextran
Kanamycin	Methoxyflurane
Cephaloridine	
Rifampicin	
Sulphonamides	

If such a regimen fails to hold the situation, then dialysis is indicated and should be started at an early stage before advanced symptoms have developed. Its aim is to prevent rather than treat complications. Specific biochemical indices usually quoted for starting dialysis are a blood urea above 33 mmol/litre, a serum creatinine above 900 μmol/litre, uncontrollable hyperkalaemia and severe metabolic acidosis, but the patient's general state is always more meaningful than a single biochemical value.

Peritoneal or haemodialysis may be used; both are suitable for the majority of patients, and when effective dialysis has been established both the fluid and the dietary restrictions can be relaxed.

Peritoneal dialysis

Peritoneal dialysis uses the peritoneum as a dialysing membrane. Waste products, water and electrolytes move across in between the plasma in the capillaries and the dialysis fluid in the peritoneal cavity. The rate and direction of movement of any substance are determined by the concentration and osmotic gradients on each side of the membrane.

Peritoneal dialysis is, practically, much simpler and cheaper to carry out than haemodialysis. The peritoneal catheter is introduced in the mid-line below the umbilicus. One or two litres of the chosen dialysis fluid are then run in and removed from the peritoneal cavity in a cyclic fashion until a satisfactory biochemical equilibrium has been achieved.

Choice of the dialysis fluid

Three kinds of dialysis fluid are available.

1. An approximately isotonic fluid (for example, Dialaflex 61).
2. A hypertonic fluid due to added glucose (for example, Dialaflex 62). These Contain sodium (141 mmol/litre), chloride (100.8 mmol/litre), calcium (1.8 mmol/litre) and magnesium (0.75 mmol/litre).
3. A fluid with a lower sodium concentration (for example, Dialaflex 63).

None of them contains potassium, which is added as the serum potassium level falls. The isotonic fluid is most commonly used because it avoids removing too much water too quickly. If, however, the patient is seriously water overloaded the hypertonic solution is used, but only for a limited time because the high glucose content (63.6 g/litre) makes it irritant to the peritoneum and also causes hyperglycaemia which may require insulin for its control.

Complications

Any of several complications may arise.

1. Perforation of a viscus during insertion of the catheter.
2. Bleeding, usually from the abdominal wali; this invariably stops spontaneously.

3. Infection of the peritoneum. The risks of this increase with the duration of the dialysis. Signs of peritonitis appear and the returning dialysis fluid becomes turbid. This fluid must be sent for culture and appropriate antibiotics given, some in the dialysis fluid.

4. Protein loss in the fluid drained from the peritoneal cavity can be considerable and may lead to hypoproteinaemia.

5. Pulmonary complications: collapse of the lung bases may occur in patients who are being ventilated.

Contraindications

These relate to mechanical problems that interfere with the flow and exchange of the dialysis fluid. They are the presence of intraperitoneal adhesions, abdominal drains or sinuses. If for such reasons peritoneal dialysis is precluded, haemodialysis will be necessary. This may be preferred as the first choice in hypercatabolic patients because the blood urea level can be controlled more readily, and when the patient is being cared for in a specialist renal unit, where the staff are familiar with the techniques involved.

Haemodialysis

Haemodialysis brings the patient's blood and the dialysing fluid to opposite sides of a semi-permeable membrane, across which the necessary exchange of water and solutes can occur. Access to the patient's circulation is usually via an arteriovenous shunt in the arm. These are created by PTFE (Teflon) tips joined by a silicone (Silastic) bridge which is removed at the time of dialysis. The patient's own blood pressure drives the blood to the machine and therefore haemodialysis may not be possible if the patient is hypotensive.

A haemodialysis unit consists of a dialysis machine and a dialyser containing the membrane. The machine controls the delivery of both the patient's blood and the dialysis fluid to the dialyser; dialysing fluid is usually premixed from a concentrate. Dialysers differ in their specifications and physical appearance, and a number of disposable models are commercially available. The shape depends upon the way the membrane is arranged, which may be as coils, flat sheets or numerous small capillary tubes—all designed to expose the circulating blood to a relatively large surface area of membrane (Fig. 20.1).

The frequency and duration of each haemodialysis are dictated by the patient's condition, but it usually requires only a few hours each day.

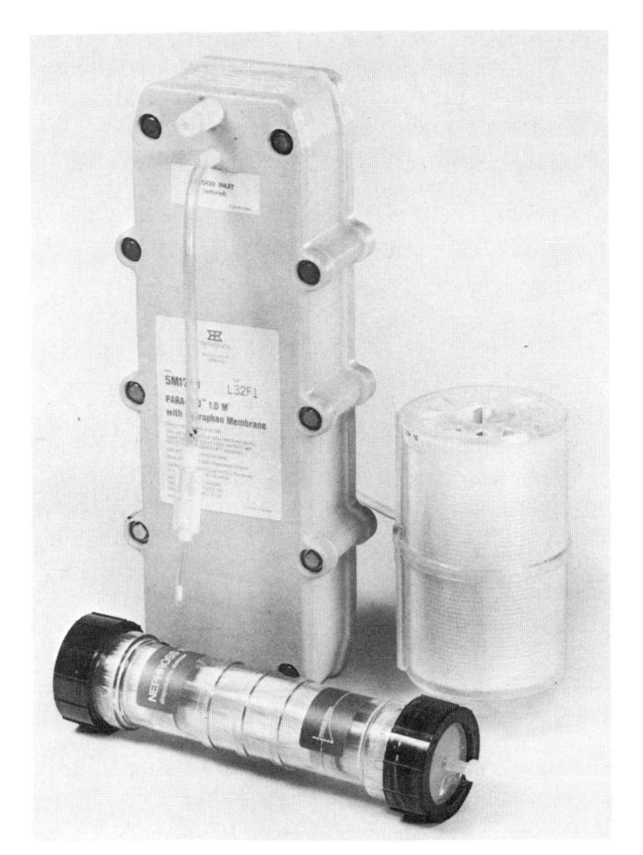

Fig. 20.1 Three dialysers.

Other measures

Anaemia should be treated with packed red blood cells. Antacid therapy or cimetidine are helpful in preventing bleeding from stress ulcers, especially in post-traumatic patients.

The recovery phase

This starts after a varying period. The urine volume increases, but the urine is initially very dilute (diuretic phase) because the kidneys are initially unable to conserve water and electrolytes. During this period vigilance must not be relaxed, for disturbances of fluid and electrolyte balance readily occur. Slowly, with the recovery of renal function, the volume and consistence of the urine return to normal. If anuria persists after three weeks of dialysis, renal biopsy should be performed to establish the pathological diagnosis. Should this reveal an irreversible condition such as cortical necrosis, the patient will have to be considered for a chronic dialysis programme and renal transplantation.

21

Fluid and electrolyte disorders

In the critically ill patient the majority of fluid and electrolyte disorders have a mixed aetiology and often more than one type is present. In this chapter they are considered separately for convenience but it is important to remember that they can coexist. Their treatment is based on an understanding of the pathophysiology and never on a 'cookery book' approach.

The terms 'hypo' and 'hyper' are used to indicate plasma levels of the electrolyte below and above the normal range for the reporting laboratory.

Water

Negative water balance—dehydration

Dehydration is a consequence of a decreased input of water, an increased output or a combination of both. Water is initially lost from the plasma. The osmolality of the plasma rises and water moves from the interstitial compartment. the latter now has a higher osmolality than the ICF and water moves out of the cells. Therefore all the fluid compartments share the total deficit.

A decreased input occurs when the patient is unable to drink or swallow for any reason.

An increased output can arise from a number of sources.

1. *The gastrointestinal tract*: vomiting, diarrhoea, nasogastric suction, or loss into the bowel as in paralytic ileus.
2. *The kidneys*: diabetes mellitus, diuretic therapy, diabetes insipidus and certain forms of renal disease.
3. *The skin*: sweating, particularly that due to a raised body temperature.
4. *The respiratory tract*: in hyperventilation of any cause.

Clinical features
These reflect the reduced ECF volume and its high osmolality. they are thirst, dry tongue and mucous membranes, loss of skin turgor, sunken eyeballs, tachycardia, low CVP and oliguria.

The urine has a high specific gravity and osmolality.

Laboratory findings
The haemoglobin level and haematocrit are raised because of the haemoconcentration and so, for the same reasons, are the blood levels of sodium, chloride and urea.

Treatment
Treatment consists of replacing the water deficit and correcting the source of abnormal loss. The water may be provided orally but in the seriously ill is best given as 5 per cent dextrose intravenously.

The presence of the clinical signs of dehyration indicate a severe degree of water depletion, at least 4 litres in a 70 kg man. During replacement at least 50 per cent of the deficit should be given in the first 24 hours. Care must be taken not to give the fluid too rapidly in patients with heart disease, to avoid the risk of precipitating pulmonary oedema.

Positive water balance—over-hydration

Overhydration increases the ECF volume.

It is often iatrogenic due to excessive fluid replacement, especially in a condition where the normal routes of excretion are affected—for instance, in renal and cardiac failure.

Clinical features
These reflect the expanded ECF volume and include sacral and peripheral oedema, pulmonary oedema and a raised CVP.

Laboratory findings
The serum sodium, osmolality and haematocrit are reduced and the urine has a low specific gravity and osmolality.

Treatment
The necessary adjustments to fluid balance must be made and diuretics given if necessary.

Sodium (normal serum level 132–145 mmol/litre)

It is important to appreciate that the serum level of sodium does not necessarily indicate the state of the total body sodium. The measured concentration reflects only the relative amounts of sodium and water present in the ECF and may not represent the overall state of sodium balance.

Hyponatraemia

This is one of the commonest electrolyte abnormalities encountered in ITU patients. It can be due either to dilution (a relative excess of water) or to sodium depletion.

In dilutional hyponatraemia, water is present in the body in excess of sodium and the total body sodium may be normal or increased. It is caused by:

1. Incorrect fluid replacement.
2. Inappropriate secretion of ADH.
3. Certain generalized disorders such as congestive heart failure and hepatic cirrhosis.

In true sodium depletion, sodium is lost is excess of water and the total body sodium and ECF are decreased. It is caused by:

1. Loss of sodium-containing fluids from the gastrointestinal tract, as in vomiting, diarrhoea or excessive nasogastric suction.
2. The use of diuretics, particularly frusemide and ethacrynic acid which increase urinary sodium loss in excess of water.

The clinical features are those of hypovolaemia.

In both forms if the serum sodium falls below 120 mmol/litre, neurological complications, due to cerebral oedema, can occur. They range from drowsiness and confusion to epileptiform convulsions and deep coma.

Treatment

If the low sodium level is due to dilution, water intake must be restricted. In true sodium depletion the sodium loss is replaced, usually with normal saline, and the abnormal source of loss corrected.

The syndrome of inappropriate ADH secretion

This syndrome is due to the continuing secretion of antidiuretic hormone (ADH) in spite of a low plasma osmolality. It is a frequent cause of hyponatraemia in the seriously ill.

Aetiology
Excess amounts of ADH or an ADH-like substance are produced, for reasons that are still not understood. It happens particularly in pulmonary and cerebral diseases, and also occurs in patients on longterm IPPV, especially when PEEP is added.

Pathophysiology
The continued high levels of ADH secretion lead to excessive water retention, and the biochemical changes are a direct result of this. The diagnosis is confirmed when the urine is found to contain large amounts of sodium and is hypertonic to plasma (that is, inappropriately concentrated).

Treatment
If the serum sodium level is above 120 mmol/litre, restriction of water intake is usually sufficient. When neurological signs are present, the water restriction has to be severe and small quantities of hypertonic saline may also be needed.

Hypernatraemia

This is a consequence of either dehydration or an excess of sodium. Over-transfusion with sodium-containing fluids (particularly sodium bicarbonate and hypertonic saline) or retention of sodium (as for instance when high doses of corticosteroids are being used) will cause an increase in body sodium. When a hypertonic solution of sodium chloride is given, the plasma osmolality increases temporarily. This stimulates ADH secretion and enhances water reabsorption from the distal tubules. Plasma osmolality returns to normal but there is an increased plasma volume. The retention of water produces the chemical picture of over-hydration and the increased blood volume may cause hypertension. The high plasma osmolality of severe hypernatraemia associated with dehydration affects the central nervous system and produces a variety of disturbances ranging from mild confusion to deep coma.

Treatment
If there is evidence of over-hydration, adjustments to sodium balance and, possibly, diuretics will be necessary. Hyperosmolality can be reduced by giving 5 per cent dextrose or hypotonic saline.

Potassium (normal serum level 3.3–4.5 mmol/litre)

Most of the body's potassium is contained in the cells and the serum level may not be representative of the total body potassium, although in general the two are related.

Hypokalaemia

Aetiology
The causes of hypokalaemia are:

1. Abnormal gastrointestinal losses due to vomiting, diarrhoea or laxative abuse.
2. Increased urinary loss, as in diabetic ketoacidosis or due to diuretic therapy.
3. Iatrogenic, due to inadequate replacement or excessive removal during peritoneal dialysis.
4. Following open-heart surgery; losses occur during cardiopulmonary bypass, and many of the patients will have been on diuretic therapy before the operation.

Clinical features
The most important effects of hypokalaemia are on the heart. Ventricular dysrhythmias occur and can progress to ventricular fibrillation. The action and toxic effects of digitalis are increased.

The ECG shows a prolonged QT interval, ST segment depression, T wave inversion and prominent U waves (positive deflections following the T wave) (Fig. 21.1).

It also effects neuromuscular function, causing muscle weakness, loss of tendon reflexes and paralytic ileus.

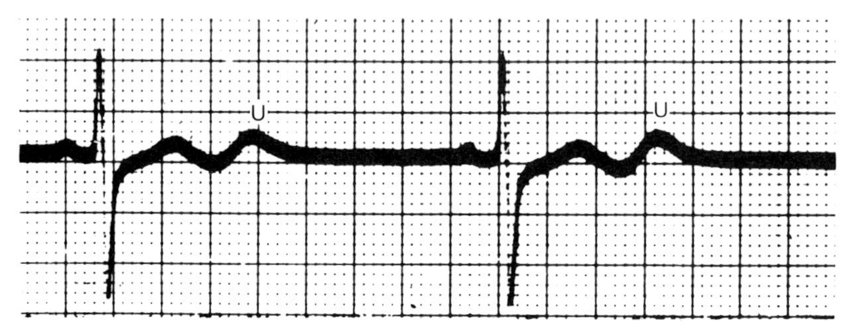

Fig. 21.1 ECG of hypokalaemia.

Treatment
Hypokalaemia requires the correction of any underlying disorder and the careful replacement of potassium (usually intravenously) at a rate, in most instances, not exceeding 10 mmol per hour. In certain cases it may have to be given more rapidly but the rate should rarely be greater than 40 mmol per hour, otherwise dangerous hyperkalaemia might ensue.

Hyperkalaemia

Aetiology

Hyperkalaemia is caused by:

1. Diminished excretion in renal failure.

2. An excess potassium load from the cells due to hypercatabolism and tissue breakdown or metabolic acidosis. If renal function is normal, however, the serum potassium will not reach dangerous levels.

3. Excess administration, either orally or intravenously; for example, massive blood transfusion.

Note that any haemolysis of the blood sample used for estimating the serum potassium spuriously increases its level in the plasma.

Clinical features

These are dominated by the effect of hyperkalaemia on the heart. As the serum potassium rises, bradycardia develops and progressively leads to dysrhythmias, heart block and cardiac arrest.

The ECG changes (Fig. 21.2) include peaking or tenting of the T waves (appears when the serum potassium is approximately 6.5 mmol/litre), widening of the QRS complex, loss of P waves and finally asystole.

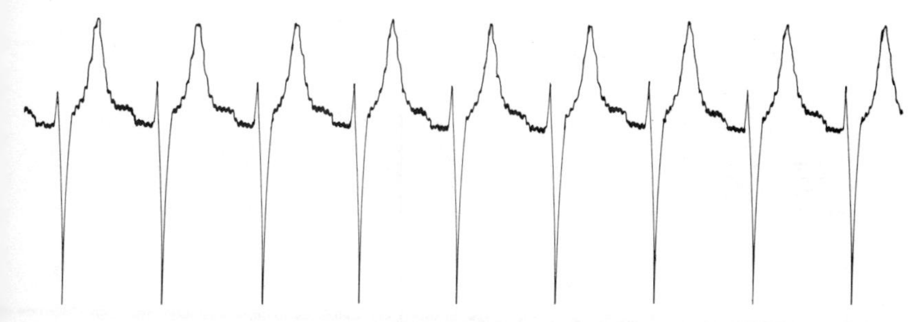

Fig. 21.2 ECG of hyperkalaemia showing peaked T waves.

Treatment

The intake of all potassium-containing solutions must be stopped. The plasma level can be lowered acutely by either of two methods, both of which move potassium into the cells.

1. Intravenous glucose and insulin (100 ml of 50 per cent glucose with 20 units of soluble insulin added).

2. Intravenous sodium bicarbonate; the creation of a metabolic alkalosis causes hydrogen ions to leave the cells in exchange for potassium ions.

The short-lived effect of these methods can be supplemented by the use of resins which exchange sodium or calcium for potassium in the bowel.

In the presence of acute renal failure and a high rate of catabolism, dialysis will inevitably be needed for continuous control of the plasma level.

General aspects of treatment

The various intravenous solutions that might be used to treat the groups of disorders that have been described are listed, together with details of their composition, in Appendix 2. In complex disorders it is better to use a number of solutions of relatively simple composition rather than one solution containing many constituents.

22

Nursing care

The nursing care of patients in acute renal failure is concerned particularly with the management of peritoneal and haemodialysis. Both techniques are widely used, but the simplicity of peritoneal dialysis makes it more readily available. In contrast, haemodialysis requires expensive specialized equipment and greater technical expertise.

Peritoneal dialysis

The nursing management of peritoneal dialysis is relatively straightforward. Various different sets of equipment are available but all consist of a disposable peritoneal catheter, a giving set and a drainage bag.

The peritoneal catheter is made of a semi-rigid plastic and has an open end and numerous small perforations near the tip. It is packaged with a removable metal stylet which acts as a guide wire during its introduction (Fig. 22.1).

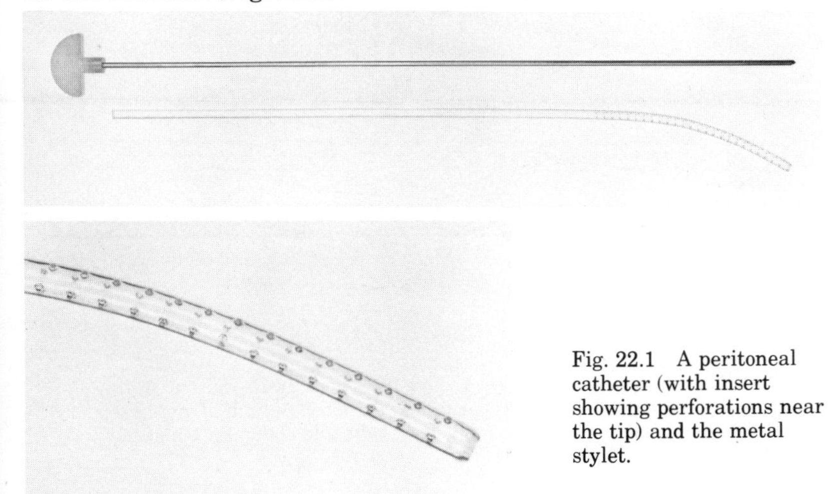

Fig. 22.1 A peritoneal catheter (with insert showing perforations near the tip) and the metal stylet.

The giving set is a double, standard type (see Fig. 22.2) giving set leading into a common drip chamber. The chamber divides into two limbs: one to the catheter and the other to the drainage bag. Control valves regulate the direction of fluid flow.

The drainage bag is calibrated, usually holding 3 litres of fluid, and has an outflow tube at the bottom.

Before use, it is essential to warm the dialysis fluid to body temperature using a thermostatically controlled warming cabinet, water tank or water bath (similar to a blood warmer). This minimizes discomfort for the patient and prevents marked changes in body temperature. The fluid's temperature must be checked before infusion by feeling the bag or bottle.

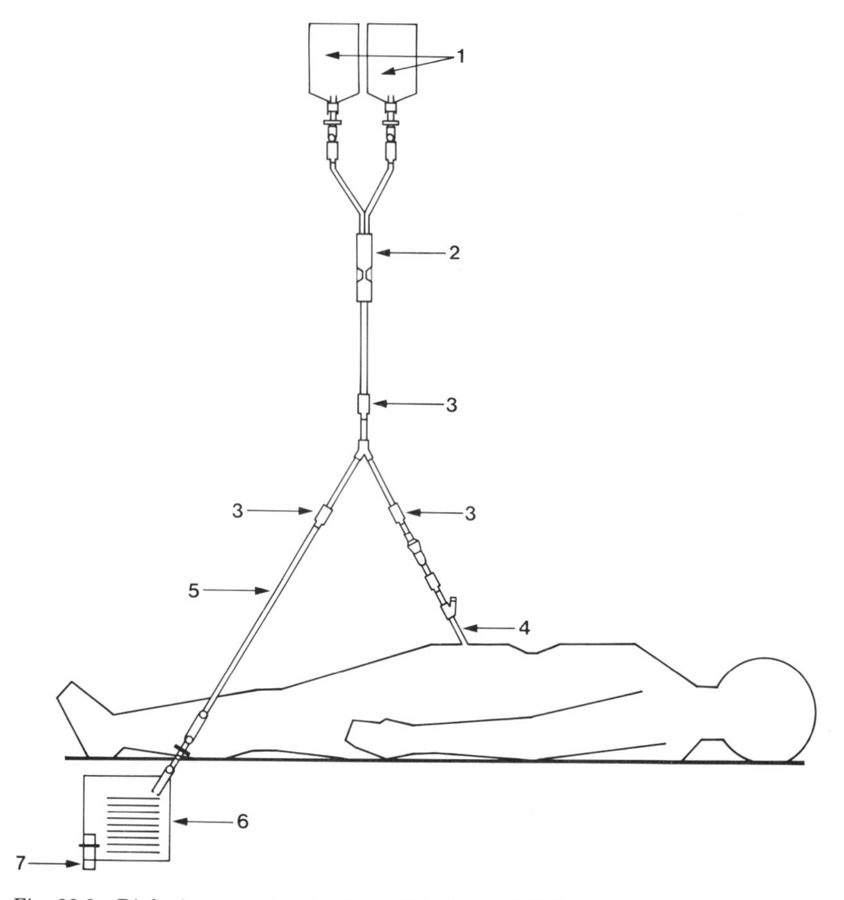

Fig. 22.2 Dialysis apparatus *in situ*: 1, litre bags of dialysis solution; 2, the giving set; 3, flow control valves; 4, peritoneal catheter; 5, limb of giving set connected to drainage bag; 6, drainage bag; 7, tube and clamp for emptying drainage bag.

Principles of management

Litre bags or bottles of warmed dialysis fluid are suspended on a drip stand and the fluid is run into the peritoneal cavity by gravity. Time is allowed for equilibration to take place across the peritoneal lining before the fluid is drained out by siphonage into the drainage bag hung below the patient's bed (Fig. 22.2).

Preparation of the patient
Explanation and reassurance are given to the conscious patient and, if possible, he is weighed. In all probability the patient will be drowsy as a result of the uraemia, but if he is concerned and apprehensive, then sedation half an hour before the insertion of the peritoneal catheter is required. The patient is asked to empty his bladder, if he is not catheterized, and the abdomen is shaved from the umbilicus to the symphysis pubis.

Insertion of the peritoneal catheter
The site selected for the insertion is usually in the mid-line one-third of the distance between the umbilicus and the symphysis pubis. Any site on the lower anterior abdominal wall may be used if operation scars have to be avoided or the catheter has to be repositioned. The mid-line is preferred since it is relatively avascular.

The operator uses a full aseptic technique and is scrubbed, gowned, gloved and masked. The abdomen is cleansed with an antiseptic solution and sterile towels are then placed around the area. Local anaesthetic (1% lignocaine) is infiltrated in the abdonimal wall down to the peritoneum. Once the area is anaesthetized, a small incision is made with a scalpel blade and the catheter is introduced. When it enters the peritoneal cavity, the metal stylet is withdrawn and the catheter advanced downwards into the pelvis.

Whilst the catheter is being introduced the nurse primes the giving set with the warmed dialysate and connects the drainage bag to the drainage limb of the set. Immediately the catheter is in place, the giving set is attached and the first dialysis cycle started. Once the solution is in the peritoneal cavity, drainage is commenced straight away. The position and patency of the catheter are established during this first cycle and only when confirmed is it stitched into position and a sterile waterproof dressing applied. Slight adjustment of the catheter may be necessary if the patient experiences pain or the solution fails to drain.

Care of the catheter involves redressing the site aseptically each day or whenever moisture leaks from around the waterproof dressing. A scrupulous technique is necessary to prevent the introduction of bacteria into the peritoneal cavity. At these times the area is observed for signs of infection—the presence of redness, swelling or tenderness.

Running the dialysis
The important objective is to maintain a 'closed' system, avoiding any unnecessary disconnection between the giving set and the catheter, or the catheter and the drainage bag, since this significantly reduces the risk of bacterial contamination. When putting up a new container of dialysis fluid, the nurse must wash her hands and then, wearing disposable gloves, swab the insertion point with an antiseptic.

The first few cycles of dialysis are carried out briskly to flush out any fibrin or blood clot in the catheter. Heparin (500 iu/litre) may be added to the early exchanges to prevent clot formation in the catheter. During the early exchanges, residual fluid may be left in the peritoneal cavity, but this is rarely of consequence because, as the exchanges progress, a negative balance is achieved.

Once the system is established, regular cycles are oganized. Each cycle consists of three stages: the run-in, the dwell and the run-out. The run-in should always be as rapid as possible and ideally 2 litres of dialysate are exchanged each hour. The sequence may be arranged as a single infusion every hour but if this volume of fluid causes the patient discomfort then litre cycles every half an hour may be more suitable.

Recording the exchanges requires a special chart which is clearly divided to show the details of each cycle (Fig. 22.3). The balance for each exchange is calculated by subtracting output from input. this will be either negative or positive and it is accordingly added to or subtracted from the cumulative balance.

THE MIDDLESEX HOSPITAL INTENSIVE THERAPY UNIT

PERITONEAL DIALYSIS

NAME [illegible]
AGE [illegible]
REG.No [illegible]

DATE 5 . 1 . 79

INSTRUCTIONS
12.00 No 62 DIAFLEX SOLN IN OVER 10 MINS & RUN OUT UNTIL STOPS.
17.00 No 62 + HEPARIN 1000u & 4 mmols KCl PER LITRE BAG.

No of Exchanges	RUN IN: TIME Start	RUN IN: TIME Finish	RUN IN: Volume	RUN IN: Type of Fluid	RUN IN: ADDITIVES	RUN OUT: TIME Start	RUN OUT: TIME Finish	RUN OUT: Volume	BALANCE This Exchange	BALANCE Daily Cumulative	REMARKS
1 / 15	12.00	12.10	1 L	No 62	NIL	12.10	13.20	1 L	–	–	
2 / 16	13.20	13.30	1 L	No 62	NIL	13.30	14.10	1 L	–	–	
3 / 17	14.10	14.20	1 L	No 62	NIL	14.20	15.40	1150	-150	-150	PINK CLEAR FLUID.
4 / 18	15.40	15.50	1 L	No 62	NIL	15.50	17.10	600	+400	+250	
5 / 19	17.10	17.20	500	No 62	HEPARIN 1000u KCl 4 mmols	17.20	18.05	800	-300	-50	
6 / 20	18.05	18.10	500	No 62	HEPARIN 1000u KCl 4 mmols	18.10	18.30	550	-50	-100	CLEARER FLUID.
7 / 21	18.30	18.40	1 L	No 62	HEPARIN 1000u KCl 4 mmols	18.40	19.15	1225	-225	-325	
8 / 22	19.15	19.25	1 L	No 62	HEPARIN 1000u KCl 4 mmols	19.25	20.05	1370	-370	-695	
9 / 23	20.05	20.15	1 L	No 62	HEPARIN 1000u KCl 4 mmols	20.15	20.50	1300	-300	-995	STRAW COLOURED FLUID
10 / 24	20.50	21.00	1 L	No 62	HEPARIN 1000u KCl 4 mmols	21.00	21.30	660	+340	-655	
11 / 25	21.30	21.45	1 L	No 62	HEPARIN 1000u KCl 4 mmols	21.45	22.15	1475	-475	-1130	CLEAR STRAW COLOURED FLUID.
12 / 26	22.15	22.25	1 L	No 62	HEPARIN 1000u KCl 4 mmols	22.25	22.55	1275	-275	-1405	

Fig. 22.3 Dialysis chart.

The volume of drainage is not constant and varies with each exchange. The drainage bag is usually calibrated, but the measurements are not always reliable and to improve accuracy the volume of drainage must be measured in a rigid calibrated container. If insufficient fluid is being removed, the drainage time may be extended, the patient's position changed to allow any fluid that might have accumulated between loops of the bowel to move, or when these manoeuvres fail a more hypertonic dialysis solution may be used.

A new dialysis chart is started every 24 hours and runs concurrently with the fluid balance chart because the totals of both charts relate to the patient's overall fluid balance.

Additives to the dialysate are absorbed via the peritoneum and must be prescribed and checked. The nurse must remember that warm dialysate is an ideal culture medium for bacteria and all additives must be made aseptically.

Common additives are:

1. Heparin (500 iu litre).
2. Potassium chloride, once hyperkalaemia has been corrected.
3. Lignocaine (50 mg/litre) to relieve pain.

Problems in running the dialysate

Failure of drainage is a common problem, with a number of possible causes: obstruction of the external tubing, excessive leakage around the catheter site, the patient's position or blockage of the catheter. The first three are simply corrected by relieving the obstruction of the tubing, inserting further sutures around the catheter or altering the patient's position. If the catheter is blocked, it is usually by fibrinous debris and should be cleared with heparinized saline, flushed several times in and out of the catheter. Should this be unsuccessful, then the catheter may be kinked inside the peritoneal cavity and minor adjustments of its position are necessary. If these measures fail, a new catheter is needed.

Pain can cause the patient great distress. It may be related to the temperature or tonicity of the dialysate. Lignocaine in the dialysate or a systemic analgestic often help. If a patient, who has previously been comfortable, complains of pain and the volume of drainage is satisfactory, infection should be suspected.

Peritonitis resulting from infected dialysis fluid, usually responds to antibiotics added to the dialysate and dialysis is not interrupted.

The features of infection are:

1. Abdominal pain, tenderness and guarding.
2. Turbidity of the drainage fluid.
3. Pyrexia.

During dialysis, samples of fluid from the catheter and drainage bag are sent each day to the laboratory for culture. This practice allows contamination to be detected at an early stage.

The incidence of infection can be minimized by following a meticulous aseptic technique in running the dialysis and when dressing the catheter site. In addition, the giving set and the drainage bag must be changed daily.

General considerations

Renal failure often occurs in association with failure of other systems. This demands all the appropriate practices of intensive therapy nursing in conjunction with the dialysis. Recording all the vital signs is essential and because fluctuations in fluid balance can occur rapidly, particularly at the beginning of dialysis, arterial pressure and central venous pressure are monitored frequently. If possible, the patient is weighed at the start of each 24 hour fluid balance period.

Once dialysis is established, fluid, salt and protein restrictions can be relaxed. Protein is lost in the fluid drained from the peritoneal cavity, which must be borne in mind when calculating the patient's nutritional needs.

Automatic cycling machines

These have several advantages. They free the nurse from repetitive tasks associated with cycling the dialysis and they reduce the incidence of infection because the system has to be 'opened' less frequently. The volume of fluid infused and the duration of each phase of the cycle can all be programmed. If the volume drained is less than the volume infused, the running out time is automatically extended. There is better temperature control and a safety device and alarm are incorporated to protect against over-heating and to denote faults in the system.

However, the machines are expensive and, in spite of their many advantages, they are probably justified only when a large-scale peritoneal dialysis programme is in operation.

Termination of dialysis

At first, dialysis is discontinued at night and recommenced during the day. Then it is completely stopped for 24 hours with the catheter left in position. Whenever dialysis is not taking place the catheter is filled with heparinized saline (to prevent blockage) and spigotted. The giving set and drainage bag are discarded and new equipment is used when dialysis is re-started.

The catheter is removed aseptically when dialysis is no longer needed. The sutures are removed, the catheter withdrawn and a sterile dressing applied. The dressing is renewed daily until the site has healed.

Haemodialysis

For haemodialysis, a permanent form of access to the circulation is required. This is usually an arteriovenous shunt placed in the arm (Fig. 22.4).

The arteriovenous shunt consists of two cannulae: one placed in an artery and the other in an adjacent vein. In between dialyses the shunt is united by a bridge (Fig. 22.4) so that blood flows from artery to vein.

Careful handling and observation of the shunt are vital if it is to last. There is an ever-present risk of infection, haemorrhage or clotting. It is this aspect of care that is the responsibility of the nurse working in an ITU, rather than the detailed technicalities of actually performing haemodialysis.

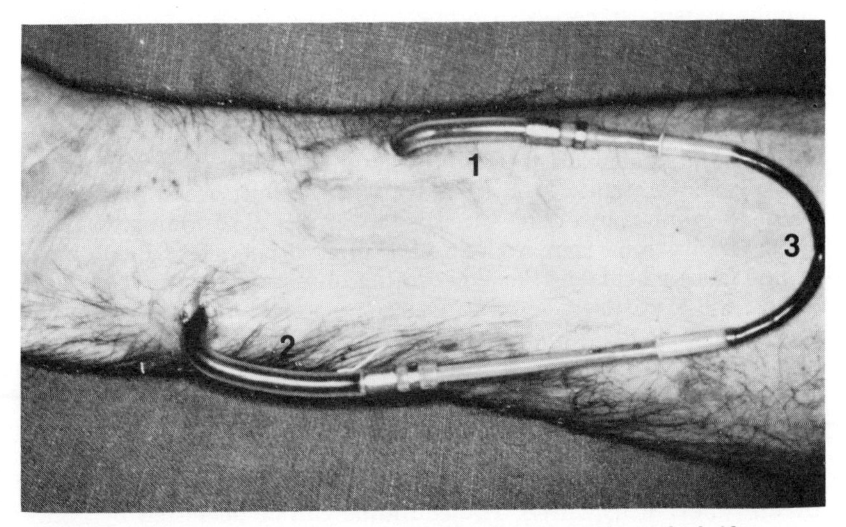

Fig. 22.4 Arteriovenous shunt: 1, arterial side; 2, venous side; 3, the bridge.

Care of the shunt

Preventing infection is extremely important and its incidence can be reduced by following a strict aseptic dressing technique and avoiding trauma to the shunt and surrounding tissues.

The shunt should be cleaned only at the beginning and end of each dialysis. Each time the dressing is taken down the area is inspected for signs of swelling, redness or the presence of a discharge—when a swab should be sent for culture. When the area has been cleansed the tubing is fixed—lighly but firmly—in position (sterile micropore tape is commonly used) so that compression, dislodgement or pulling cannot occur. The shunt is always dressed leaving a section of the bridge exposed for observation. If a bandage is used to secure the dressing, it should not be fastened with a safety pin in case the shunt is accidentally punctured.

Haemorrhage is most likely to occur when the shunt is infected, and firm pressure is usually sufficient to control the bleeding. Rapid profuse bleeding will occur if the bridge falls apart from either the arterial or the venous side of the shunt. This crisis requires prompt clamping of the arterial and venous sides of the shunt, and reconnection of the bridge. Two clamps must always be available at the bedside for this purpose.

Clotting of the shunt in between haemodialyses may be the result of construction from too tight a bandage holding the dressing in place, taking the blood pressure in the same arm as the shunt or giving drugs through the venous side of the cannula which can lead to venous spasm. It can also occur from trauma, infection or from hypotension, which is perhaps the most common cause in ITU patients.

The nurse must frequently observe the exposed section of the bridge to ensure that the blood is flowing satisfactorily through the shunt. In addition, she needs to listen for the characteristic murmur in the vein, which is readily heard with a stethoscope placed just above the venous insertion site. Disappearance of this murmur is one of the indications that a clot is forming. Other signs include the bridge feeling cold, the blood becoming blue instead of bright red in colour and eventually separating into plasma and red cell layers. If any of these signs is apparent, blood clot formation must be suspected and removal attempted urgently in order to preserve the shunt. The only exception to this would be when a shunt is infected, because of the danger of haemorrhage and the introduction of a septic embolus into the circulation.

Declotting of a shunt is a sterile procedure and must be carried out by an experienced nurse. The cannulae can be declotted by gentle suction using a syringe or by irrigation with heparinized saline. The clot must not be dislodged into the circulation because of the risks of venous or arterial embolism.

Hepatitis associated with haemodialysis

The incidence of spasmodic outbreaks, amongst staff and patients, of serum hepatitis has increased with the use of haemodialysis for the treatment of chronic renal failure. There is, however, no evidence to suggest a hepatitis problem in patients receiving haemodialysis for acute renal failure. Such patients may be carriers of the virus and must all be screened for hepatitis B (Australia) antigen before haemodialysis is started. Patients in whom this is positive must be segregated with their own dialyser.

23

Metabolic disorders

A number of diseases cause acute and severe derangements of normal metabolic function. They have widespread systemic effects which, if not controlled, can quickly lead to coma and death. Acute hepatic failure, diabetic ketoacidosis, hyperosmolar coma, and accidental hypothermia may require intensive therapy. They are described in this chapter.

Acute hepatic failure

The liver carries out a large number of vital physiological functions concerned with protein and carbohydrate metabolism. bilirubin excretion and blood coagulation. All are affected in acute liver failure.

Aetiology

Severe liver damage, sufficient to produce failure of its function, may be caused by infections, toxins or ischaemia; the commonest are;

1. Acute viral hepatitis, due either to the A or B hepatitis virus.
2. Acute poisoning with paracetamol and following halothane anaesthesia.
3. States of low cardiac output.

Clinical picture

The clinical features of liver failure are virtually the same irrespective of the aetiology, and reflect impairment of its normal functions.

1. *Jaundice* due to failure of bilirubin excretion.
2. *Encephalopathy* (hepatic coma) due to failure of the liver to remove nitrogen-containing compounds derived from protein

metabolism and from bacterial breakdown of protein in the bowel. This increases the blood levels of certain amino acids and ammonia which affect cerebral function. In addition, the liver glycogen stores are depleted and hypoglycaemia occurs. This and associated disturbances of electrolytes and blood gas tensions aggravate the coma. According to its severity, hepatic coma is graded into four stages:

I. The patient is confused and often very agitated.
II. The degree of confusion is more marked and a flapping tremor of the hands and feet may be present. The EEG becomes abnormal in this stage and remains so in stages III and IV.
III. The patient is more deeply comatose but still rousable.
IV. Deep coma is present and there may be respiratory and circulatory disturbances due to cerebral oedema.

3. *Abnormal bleeding tendency* due to a combination of impaired synthesis of clotting factors, thrombocytopenia and abnormal platelet function. Haemorrhage can occur spontaneously at any site, especially into the skin and gastrointestinal tract.

4. *Ascites and oedema* are both the result of hypoproteinaemia from failure of the liver to synthesize albumin.

The patients are also more susceptible to bacteraemia and more likely to develop acute renal failure.

Biochemical changes

High levels of transaminase enzymes (SGOT and SGPT) in the blood indicate the severity of the liver cell damage. The serum bilirubin is increased and the plasma proteins and blood glucose are decreased. Tests of blood coagulation are abnormal.

The blood must be screened for hepatitis B (Australia) antigen which will be present in cases of acute hepatitis due to the B virus.

Treatment

If viral hepatitis is suspected, the patient must be isolated. Particular emphasis should be placed on the infectivity of blood, saliva, urine and stools, and these must be handled with great care.

The liver has remarkable powers of regeneration and the aim of treatment is to correct the toxic and metabolic disturbances and to maintain vital functions to provide sufficient time for this to take place.

It is essential to:

1. Clear and sterilize the bowel contents to prevent absorption of protein breakdown products. This is accomplished with frequent magnesium sulphate enemas, oral neomycin (4–8 g per day) to reduce the bacterial flora and lactulose (30 ml eight-hourly) which is

thought to act by trapping ammonia in the bowel. No protein at all is allowed in the diet.

2. Withold any sedative drugs, even if the patient is very restless. They are all potentially dangerous and are likely to precipitate or deepen coma.

3. Correct hypoglycaemia with 10 per cent or higher concentrations of dextrose intravenously and maintain meticulous fluid and electrolyte balance.

4. Correct the coagulation disorders with fresh frozen plasma. Vitamin K is given but has a limited effect when severe liver damage is present. Cimetidine, a histamine-blocking drug (H_2 antagonist), is given routinely to reduce gastric acidity and minimize the risks of gastric bleeding.

5. Treat bacteraemia and failure in other systems, particularly renal and respiratory, as and when they arise. Sudden and unexpected respiratory arrest may occur, and facility for immediate ventilation must be at hand.

A number of other measures have been tried—some dramatic—but they have had little effect on the overall mortality and have been abandoned. All were aimed at removing from the blood those substances (many of which are still unidentified) responsible for causing the coma. They have included dialysis, exchange transfusions, cross-circulation with human volunteers or non-human primates and haemoperfusion through charcoal columns.

Steroids are often given but have no proven value, except in the treatment of cerebral oedema, and can cause additional complications.

Prognosis

This depends on the extent of the liver damage as clinically reflected by the severity of the encephalopathy. About 75 per cent of patients in stages I–III can be expected to survive but in stage IV this figure falls dramatically to around 10 per cent. Death may be due solely to the hepatic failure or to cerebral oedema, gastrointestinal haemorrhage or sepsis.

Diabetic ketoacidosis

This is usually a complication of established diabetes, commonly precipitated by an intercurrent infection or other acute medical or surgical illness that increases the requirements for insulin. Occasionally it is the presenting feature of diabetes.

The underlying biochemical disturbance is an absolute or relative deficiency of insulin. As a consequence, glucose is not utilized by the tissues, hyperglycaemia develops and glucose 'spills over' into the urine. This glycosuria causes an osmotic diuresis with large losses of water, salt and potassium, and leads to severe dehydration and electrolyte disturbances.

The body attempts to compensate for the diminished glucose uptake by breaking down adipose tissue to meet energy needs. The excessive breakdown of fats leads to an accumulaiton of keto acids (acetoacetic and hydroxybutyric acid) in the blood and their appearance in the urine (ketonuria). They produce a metabolic acidosis which stimulates the respiratory centre and the patient hyperventilates.

The two major disturbances of insulin deficiency are, therefore, hyperglycaemia and ketoacidosis.

Clinical features

These relate to the biochemical abnormalities and include thirst, polyuria, hyperventilation (Kussmaul breathing or 'air hunger') and an altered state of consciousness. The patients are severely dehydrated with a tachycardia and hypotension. The smell of acetone may be detectable in the breath and there may be an obvious site of infection.

Biochemical findings

In the blood there is a high glucose level around 30–35 mmol/litre, a low potassium and a metabolic acidosis. The urine contains glucose and ketone bodies.

Blood, urine and sputum samples should be sent for culture, and swabs taken from any infected skin lesions and also from the throat if it appears inflamed.

Treatment

Insulin, intravenous fluids and potassium are given and any underlying infection is treated with antibiotics.

If possible, neither a CVP line nor a urinary catheter should be inserted because of the risks of introducing infection.

Soluble insulin. There are many different regimens for giving insulin; the following reflects the author's preference. It should be continuously infused intravenously—ideally by a constant infusion pump, but if one of these is not available it may be added to a burette. The starting dose is 10 units per hour and the blood glucose is measured each hour. If this dose fails to reduce the level, it is increased to 20 units per hour, but if the glucose has fallen below 16 mmol/litre it is reduced to 5 units per hour. It should be possible to change to subcutaneous insulin after 48 hours.

Intravenous fluids. Normal saline is given initially at a rate of 500 ml per hour for two to four hours and then at 250 ml per hour until the blood sugar is below 16 mmol/litre, when it is changed to 5 per cent dextrose. Plasma may be necessary in severely hypotensive patients.

Potassium is replaced according to the level of the serum potassium, which should be measured hourly. The metabolic acidosis usually disappears as the hyperglycaemia is corrected and circulation improves; sodium bicarbonate is required only occasionally.

With these measures, the mortality for diabetic ketoacidosis has fallen to around 5 per cent.

Hyperosmolar coma

This occurs mainly in elderly diabetics who may have other serious medical disorders. There is a very high blood glucose (50–60 mmol/litre) but no ketoacidosis. The main clinical features are impairment of consciousness and severe dehydration. Less insulin is required than in diabetic ketoacidosis and the hyperosmolar state is treated with 0.5 normal saline.

Accidental hypothermia

Unintentional or accidental hypothermia can occur at any age, but is commonest in the elderly whose means of temperature regulation are impaired by various acute or chronic diseases, or drugs, and who often live alone in inadequately heated accommodation. Fit adults have normal thermoregulation but this can be rendered ineffective by prolonged exposure to severe cold.

A patient is described as hypothermic if the central (rectal) temperature is less than 35°C, and severely so if it is less than 32°C.

Clinical features

The skin feels like that of a corpse and the limbs are pale and cyanosed, sometimes with incipient gangrene of the fingers and toes. The mental state depends on the degree of hypothermia and ranges from confusion to coma. There is cardiorespiratory depression with bradycardia, hypotension and slow shallow breathing.

Hypoglycaemia is frequent and the ECG characteristically shows sinus bradycardia and the presence of J waves, positive deflections at the junction of the QRS and ST segments (Fig. 23.1).

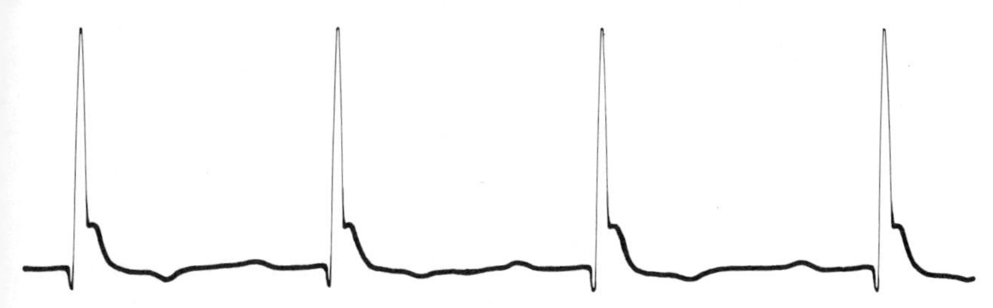

Fig. 23.1 ECG in hypothermia, showing J waves.

Treatment

Patients with severe hypothermia are best treated in an ITU. The body temperature is continuously monitored and gradually increased (0.5°C per hour) by nursing the patient in a warm room and using a 'space' blanket, supplemented, if necessary, by IPPV with warm (37°C) humidified air. Varying degrees of failure are invariably present in all systems and these are treated in the usual manner. The value of steroids is debatable.

All elderly patients who recover should be seen by a social worker before they are discharged from hospital, to ensure that their living circumstances are adequate to prevent a further episode of hypothermia.

24
Acute poisoning

The incidence of acute poisoning has increased dramatically during the past 20 years. The major increase has been in intentional self-poisoning, which now accounts for about 15 per cent of all admissions to acute medical wards, the more serious of which require intensive therapy. It is commonest between the ages of 15 and 25 years and more frequent in females.

A wide variety of drugs are taken by patients intent on self-poisoning, the pattern reflecting the kinds of drugs that are readily available at a particular time. Increasingly, several are taken together and often in combination with alcohol.

The most commonly used are the barbiturate and non-barbiturate hypnotics, the benzoidazepines, tricyclic antidepressants, salicylates and paracetamol, but each year, as new compounds appear, the 'league table' changes.

Diagnosis

In spite of many drugs that can be taken, the clinical features, with a few notable exceptions, are not dissimilar. A history is all important; conscious patients usually provide all the necessary information and when the patient is unconscious accounts from relatives or friends can be very helpful. If a diagnosis of acute poisoning is suspected, it is then necessary to identify the poisons and assess the quantity and time at which they were taken.

In general, the rather non-specific clinical picture of varying degrees of coma is of little help in identifying the poisons. Exceptions are the characteristic features of salicylate poisoning, the smell of coal gas on the breath in carbon monoxide poisoning, and the pin-point pupils caused by opiates. Skin bullae (large blisters surrounded by a rim of erythema) occur mainly in severe barbiturate poisoning but are not entirely specific. They are found on pressure areas between opposing skin surfaces such as the inner aspects of the knees and ankles. Injection marks around veins and the presence of superficial necrotic ulcers point to 'mainline' drug addiction.

Laboratory identification of the poison

The chemical analysis of samples of blood, urine or gastric aspirate can provide positive identification of the poisons and measurement of blood levels is a guide to the quantity taken. In some cases the use of this service is essential for proper patient management but it must be recognized that very few specific antidotes exist. Knowledge of the quantities of drug present in the blood is rarely helpful in the initial treatment except in the case of salicylates and paracetamol; many of the laboratory methods are difficult and lengthy. Consequently, all requests need to be carefully considered if the service is not to be abused. The various samples should always be collected—if only for medicolegal reasons—and stored if immediate analysis is not deemed necessary.

Clinical assessment of the severity of poisoning

The majority of drugs that are taken affect the patient's level of consciousness, and as a consequence coma of varying degree frequently dominates the clinical picture. The other systems are also involved, sometimes to a greater extent than the central nervous system, and all cases require a full systematic clinical assessment.

Central nervous system

The level of coma is graded and the state of the pupillary and peripheral reflexes noted.

Respiratory system.

The important features are the vulnerability of the airway and the adequacy of ventilation. The protective pharyngeal 'gag' reflexes are tested and the rate, depth and pattern of respiration measured. A respiratory rate of less than 10 per minute and a minute volume of less than 4 litres per minute indicate serious respiratory depression.

Cardiovascular system

Dysrhythmias, shock and dehydration may all be present in severe cases. Hypothermia is often related to the severity of the condition and can be severe in patients who have been unconscious for a long period of time in an exposed situation. The significance of skin bullae has already been mentioned.

Management

Important advances in treatment have occurred during the past 20 years. With the introduction of the various methods of intensive care the mortality of acute barbiturate poisoning, for example, has fallen from 25 per cent to less than 1 per cent.

Emergency treatment

This is carried out in the admission room and consists of resuscitative measures and adopting means to prevent any further absorption of the poison.

Establishing and maintaining a clear airway is of paramount importance. Any debris, vomitus or displaced dentures are removed from the mouth and upper airways, and if the cough and gag reflexes are depressed an oropharyngeal airway is inserted. Deeply comatose patients should be intubated.

In an effort to prevent further absorption of the poison, the stomach can be emptied by inducing vomiting or by gastric lavage. Both of these methods are potentially hazardous and should never be undertaken lightly. The induction of vomiting is contemplated only if the patient is fully conscious, when stimulation of the pharynx with a finger, spoon or spatula is usually effective. Emetics should not be given; they take time to act and meanwhile the patient's level of consciousness may deteriorate so that, when vomiting eventually occurs, there is a considerable risk of aspiration.

Gastric lavage can also lead to the aspiration of gastric contents and the airway must be intact or protected before it is used. Its value is in any case limited and it is unlikely to be of value if more than four hours have elapsed since the poison was taken, except in the case of salicylate poisoning. It is absolutely contraindicated after the ingestion of caustic or corrosive poisons.

Intensive therapy

Support of the various systems, along the lines outlined in the previous chapters, is the mainstay of treatment. Respiratory failure, cardiovascular failure, fluid and electrolyte disturbances, and hypothermia may all be present in severe cases.

The basic methods of intensive therapy are supplemented in certain cases by techniques that hasten the elimination of the poison.

Forced diuresis

This is used for drugs that are excreted predominantly in the urine. Large volumes of alkaline or acidic fluids are given to promote a diuresis. The pH of the urine determines the solubility of the particular drug. Meticulous management of fluid balance is essential when carrying out any form of forced diuresis.

Alkaline diuresis

This is effective in severe salicylate poisoning. Five hundred ml of 5 per cent dextrose, 0.9 per cent saline and 1.26 per cent sodium bicarbonate are each given intravenously in rotation at an overall rate of 2 litres per hour. Potassium supplements are necessary and diuretics can be given to increase the urine volume. The pH of the urine should be measured frequently and should be 7.5 or above (a pH of 8 is the physiological upper limit of urinary pH).

Acid diuresis

Ammonium chloride is used instead of sodium bicarbonate to achieve a urinary pH below 7. It is advocated in severe amphetamine poisoning but is seldom used.

Dialysis

Both peritoneal and haemodialysis can be used but their role is limited and they should be considered only if progressive clinical deterioration occurs despite full supportive care.

Haemoperfusion

By passing the patient's blood through columns of charcoal or other exchange resins, certain poisons—especially barbiturates and glutethimide—can be removed. At the present time it has a very limited place in management, the indications being similar to those for dialysis.

After-care

When the patient recovers consciousness, there may be extreme restlessness and, in the case of alcoholics and chronic drug addicts, delirium tremens can occur.

Psychiatric treatment

The management of patients with self-poisoning is incomplete without psychiatric consultation, and this must be arranged whilst the patient is in the ITU. The size or severity of the overdose bears no relation to the underlying degree of mental instability. Many such patients are remorseful, depressed and anxious, and require a great degree of support from the nursing staff.

25
Coma

'Coma' comes from the Greek, *koma*, meaning deep sleep. The word is used here to describe any state of impaired consciousness, regardless of its aetiology.

Between normal awareness and deep, unresponsive, coma there are many different levels of conscious impairment. These form a continuum, merging one into another, not a series of discrete steps or clinical grades. Unfortunately, many of the classifications of coma, that are in clinical use, are based on a false assumption that clearly defined levels do exist. They have created a confused, and often ambiguous, set of terms; descriptions such as 'light coma', 'moderate coma', 'drowsy', 'a bit deeper' are commonly used, but are rather meaningless except to the person using them. Their use should be banned from the bedside recording of neurological observations and replaced by an objective record of the state of the patient, defining responses of specific stimuli. Such a scheme has been adopted in the Glasgow Coma Scale (described later), which enables quantitative measurements and meaningful comparisons to be made.

Causes of coma

A normal state of consciousness requires integration of function between the cerebral cortex and the reticular formation in the brain stem. The conditions that lead to coma affect these structures either separately or in combination. The cortex has to be diffusely affected whereas the reticular formation can be interrupted by relatively localized lesions.

The causes of coma are many, but they can be placed into two groups: intrinsic, occurring within the brain, and extrinsic, arising as a result of disturbances in other systems (Table 25.1). Cerebral oedema is often a feature, and in some instances herniation (coning) of the brain causes a rapid deterioration of neurological function.

Table 25.1 The cause of coma

Intrinsic	Extrinsic
Cerebrovascular lesions:	Metabolic disorders:
Subarachnoid haemorrhage	Anoxia
Intracerebral haemorrhage	Hypercapnia
Cerebral thrombosis and embolism	Hyperglycaemia
	Ketoacidosis
Space-occupying lesions:	Uraemia
Cerebral tumour	Hepatic failure
Cerebral abscess	
Extradural haematoma	Drugs
Subdural haematoma	
	Endocrine disturbances:
Head injury	Myxoedema
	Hypopituitarism
Meningitis and encephalitis	

Cerebral oedema

Many of the processes which cause coma also cause cerebral oedema and it is often this that disturbs cerebral function.

Pathogenesis

Cerebral hypoxia, inflammation of the brain and meninges, cerebral trauma and systemic metabolic disturbances all increase the permeability of the brain capillaries; as a result there is an increase in both the intra- and extracellular water content of the brain—which is cerebral oedema.

Effects on cerebral function

Because of its increased water content, the brain swells within the rigid encasement of the skull and there is a rise in intracranial pressure. This impedes cerebral blood flow and aggravates the situation, resulting in a vicious circle.

The distribution of the oedema fluid is not necessarily uniform, and variations of pressure may occur within the brain substance itself. These will produce shifts and distortion of the brain and might result in herniation (coning) of certain structures through the tentorial opening or the foramen magnum. Such an event causes deformity and ischaemia of the brain stem and leads to a rapid deterioration of consciousness with failure of vital functions.

Treatment

Treatment constitutes an extremely important part of the management of many comatose patients. Its aim is to reduce the elevated intracranial pressure, correct the distortions of brain tissue and improve cerebral blood flow.

1. *Steroids.* Dexamethasone reduces the water content of the brain and is given in an initial dose of 10 mg intravenously followed by 4 mg six-hourly.

2. *Hypertonic solutions and diuretics.* Mannitol (20 per cent solution) or frusemide are used; they have a quicker action than dexamethasone, but are less effective. The main indication for their use is in the emergency treatment of acute herniation.

3. *Hyperventilation.* Lowering the arterial P_{CO_2} to 25 mmHg (3.3 kPa) by IPPV causes cerebral vasoconstriction and reduces the bulk of the intracranial contents, and so lowers intracranial pressure. It is most helpful after extensive neurosurgery and in patients with serious head injuries.

Herniation (coning)

In any intracranial disorder, herniation or coning of brain tissue causes a rapid worsening of coma and a disturbance of brain stem function. It occurs in association with severe cerebral oedema, massive cerebral haemorrhage, encephalitis, cerebral tumours and extradural haematomas. With a rise in pressure in the anterior fossa of the skull, parts of the cerebral hemispheres are forced through the tentorial opening into the posterior fossa. Progression of this process may then cause the cerebellum to herniate through the foramen magnum.

The clinical manifestations of coning are:

1. Deterioration in conscious level.

2. Dilatation of the pupil and loss of the pupillary light reflex because of kinking of the third cranial (oculomotor) nerve. This may happen on one or both sides, depending on the position of the herniation.

3. Increased tone in the limbs.

4. Respiratory dysfunction; changes in respiratory rate and rhythm are danger signs and respiratory arrest may develop suddenly.

5. Arterial hypertension and bradycardia are less constant features.

Assessing an unconscious patient

Observations on the neurological status of a comatose patient must include objective details of the level of coma and indices of the function of the cerebral cortex and brain stem.

The deficiencies of the many different systems used for this purpose have already been mentioned. They provide no clear guidance of what should be noted and encourage free-hand description with all its known imperfections.

The Glasgow Coma Scale (Fig. 25.1)

The Glasgow Coma Scale overcomes the drawbacks mentioned above. It describes the states of impaired consciousness by detailing three aspects of behavioural response that can be formally tested and recorded in a standardized, repeatable manner. They are eye opening, verbal response and motor response, each of which is evaluated independently of the others. The results are then graded and can be represented graphically over a period of time.

Eye opening

1. *Spontaneous*: whilst this indicates arousal, it does not necessarily mean that the patient is aware of his surroundings. Even what appear to be purposive, following, eye movements can be of a reflex nature.
2. *In response to speech and to pain*: These are self-explanatory.

Verbal response

The content of speech is graded as:

1. *Orientated*: the patient responds to conversation and shows himself to be normally aware and orientated in time and place.
2. *Confused*: the response to conversation is confused and shows various degrees of disorientation.
3. *Inappropriate*: speech occurs sporadically, occasionally as shouting. The utterances are often unintelligible and not in response to conversational stimuli.
4. *Incomprehensible*: this refers to moaning and groaning without any recognizable words.

These verbal responses cannot, of course, be tested in patients who are intubated or have a tracheostomy and this is indicated on the chart.

Motor response

The ability to obey commands is the best response possible. When eliciting this the nurse must always be aware of certain reflex movements, such as the grasp reflex, that may mimic voluntary responses.

Form No. M127

THE MIDDLESEX HOSPITAL INTENSIVE THERAPY UNIT

NEUROLOGICAL OBSERVATION CHART

SURNAME ....
FIRST NAMES ....

REG No ....
DATE OF BIRTH ....

DATE .... TIME: 12 noon, 30, 13.00, 30, 14.00, 30, 15.00, 30, 16.00, 30, 17.00, 30, 18.00, 30, 19.00, 30, 20.00, 30, 21.00, 30, 22.00, 30, 23.00, 30, 24.00, 30, 01.00, 30, 02.00, 30, 03.00, 30, 04.00, 30, 05.00, 30, 06.00, 30, 07.00, 30, 08.00, 30, 09.00, 30, 10.00, 30, 11.00, 30

			Notes
COMA SCALE	Eyes open	Spontaneously	Eyes closed by swelling = c
		To speech	
		To pain	
		None	
	Best verbal response	Orientated	Endotracheal tube or tracheostomy = T
		Confused	
		Inappropriate	
		Incomprehensible	
		None	
	Best motor response	Obey commands	Usually record the best arm response
		Localize pain	
		Flexion to pain	
		Extension to pain	
		None	
PUPILS	+ reacts − no reaction c eye closed	R Size	Size R
		R Reaction	Reaction R
		L Size	Size L
		L Reaction	Reaction L
PATTERN OF LIMB MOVEMENTS Score 1-5 as below	R	Arm	Arm R
		Leg	Leg R
	L	Arm	Arm L
		Leg	Leg L

1, 2, 3 record differences in strength between limbs with movements better than types 4 and 5. 1 - normal strength. 2 - weakness.
When R and L limbs are both weak but to different degrees, then 3 - weakest side. 4 - spastic/abnormal flexion. 5 - extension.

PUPIL SCALE: 1 mm, 2 mm, 3 mm, 4 mm, 5 mm, 6 mm, 7 mm, 8 mm

SHEET No ....

Fig. 25.1 The Glasgow Coma Scale.

Where there is no response to verbal command, a standarized painful stimulus—in the upper limbs, pressure on the nail bed using a pencil, and in the lower limbs, compression of the Achilles tendon between thumb and forefinger—is applied. Pinching the skin or rubbing the sternum with a clenched fist are not only disfiguring but unnecessary.

The responses to painful stimulation are:

1. *Localized*: the patient attempts to voluntarily withdraw the stimulated limb.

2. *Flexor*: there is reflex flexion of the tested limb and often of the other limbs.

3 *Extensor posturing*: there is extension of some of the limbs. The two classic forms described are decorticate and decerebrate rigidity.

(a) Decorticate rigidity (Fig. 25.2a) consists of flexion of the arms, wrists and fingers with extension of the legs; it signifies interruption of the corticospinal tracts in the cerebral hemispheres. It may also be provoked by tracheal suction.

(b) Decerebrate rigidity (Fig. 25.2b) consists of arching of the back and rigid extension of the arms and legs, sometimes accompanied by hyperpnoea; it indicates the presence of damage to the cerebral hemispheres and upper brain stem (mid-brain and pons).

4. *No response*: this is usually associated with flaccidity of the limbs, but before recording this always check that the stimulus is adequate and test both sides.

Grading coma in this way provides an indication of overall cerebral impairment, and is followed by a more specific examination of brain stem function. Considerable information about this is obtained from examination of the pupils, certain reflex eye movements and the pattern of respiration.

State of the pupils

The normal size of the pupil is governed by a balance of activity between the parasympathetic and the sympathetic nerve supplies to the pupillary sphincter muscle, the dominance of one over the other depending on the level of illumination and other factors. An increase in sympathetic activity dilates the pupils and an increase in parasympathetic activity constricts it. If both are damaged, the sphincter muscle relaxes and the pupil is dilated.

Anatomical pathways

The parasympathetic nerve supply arises in the mid-brain from a small nucleus adjacent to the third nerve nucleus and its fibres pass to the pupil in the third nerve. The sympathetic nerves have a more indirect course: they start in the hypothalamus, pass down the brain

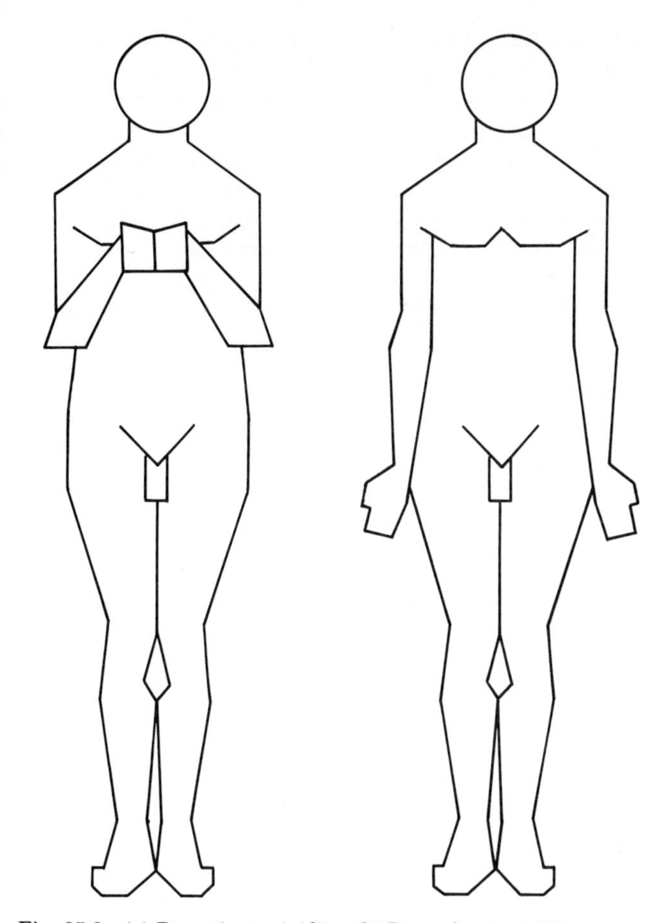

Fig. 25.2 (a) Decorticate rigidity. (b) Decerebrate rigidity.

stem and leave the spinal cord from its upper thoracic segments. They then re-enter the skull beside the internal carotid artery and reach the eye along with the ophthalmic artery.

The pathway for the pupillary light reflex is from the retina, along the optic nerve to the parasympathetic nucleus in the mid-brain (afferent), returning to the pupil along the third nerve (efferent).

Abnormalities of pupil size

One or both pupils may be affected, depending on whether the cause is unilateral or bilateral.

Dilatation occurs when the parasympathetic nerve supply is affected by lesions of the brain stem or third nerve.

Cerebral anoxia, as after a cardiac arrest, dilates both pupils and if they remain dilated for more than a few minutes this usually implies severe, probably irreversible, brain damage. Resuscitation should, however, never be abandoned on this finding alone.

Herniation of the brain through the tentorial opening damages the third nerve and the pupil dilates—initially on one side but, as the herniation increases in size, the other side is also affected.

Constriction occurs when the sympathetic nerves are damaged, as for instance by a lesion in the pons, which affects both pupils, or by a lesion in the neck, which affects only one side (Horner's syndrome).

Effect of drugs on the pupil

Many drugs used in the treatment of seriously ill patients affect the pupils; caution is thus necessary when interpreting the cause of pupil size in comatose patients receiving any of these. Atropine, by blocking the parasympathetic nerve endings, dilates the pupils and the sympathomimetic drugs, adrenaline and isoprenaline, by stimulating the sympathetic nerve endings, dilate them. The opiates, morphine and diamorphine, constrict the pupils because of their cholinergic action.

Loss of the light reflex

Normally both pupils constrict in response to a light shone into one eye. The non-stimulated pupil responds because there are interconnections between the parasympathetic nuclei of both sides. When testing this reflex a bright light must always be used; the poor light of a small torch with a failing battery is totally inadequate.

Absence of the light reflex can be due to interruption of the reflex arc anywhere along its course, afferent or efferent. In comatose patients, however, the cause almost always lies in the mid-brain or the third nerve. The pupils are non-reacting (fixed) and dilated.

Reaction to light should be recorded as present or absent and the size of the pupils measured in millimetres.

Eyelid and eye movements

Certain reflex movements of the eyelids and eyes are used to test the integrity of the brain stem.

Corneal reflex

Touching the cornea with a piece of cotton wool produces closure of the eyelids and upward movement of the eyes. Its presence indicates normal function of the brain stem between the fifth nerve nucleus (afferent), the third nerve nucleus (supplying the eye muscles) and the seventh nerve nucleus (supplying the muscles of the eyelid).

Oculocephalic reflex (doll's head phenomenon) (Fig. 25.3a)
The eyelids are held open and the head is rotated from side to side. A positive response is indicated by the eyes moving in the opposite direction to that of the rotation.

Its presence indicates intact brain stem function between the eighth cranial nerve (vestibular) and the nerves (third, fourth and sixth) supplying the eye muscles. It can also be tested in a vertical direction by extending and flexing the neck. The afferent impulses arise from the vestibular apparatus in the inner ear.

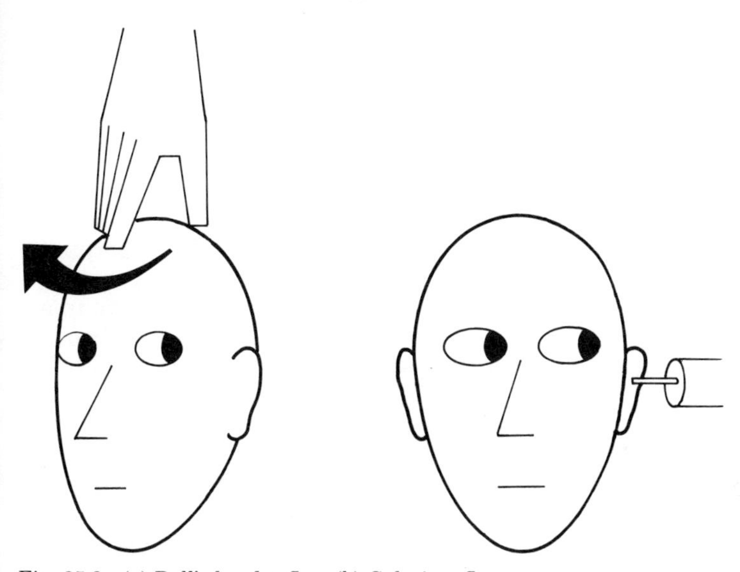

Fig. 25.3 (a) Doll's head reflex. (b) Caloric reflex.

Caloric reflex (Fig. 25.3b)
The eyelids are held open and 20 ml of ice-cold water is syringed into the ear on one side. A positive response is indicated by diversion of the eyes towards that ear. After an interval of five minutes the other side is tested.

Presence of the reflex indicates intact brain stem function over an area similar to that of the oculocephalic reflex. The afferent impulses for this reflex originate from convection currents set up in the vestibular canals.

These three reflexes give a better indication of the integrity of the brain stem over a greater area than does the pupillary light reflex. In metabolic coma they are affected earlier than the pupillary reflex, so the presence of the latter alone is of value in making a diagnosis between an intrinsic and extrinsic cause of the coma.

Cough and gag reflexes

These are provoked by stimulating the pharynx and upper respiratory tract with a spatula or catheter; normally the patient 'gags' or coughs they are essential protective reflexes, and their absence in deep coma means that the airway is vulnerable to aspiration and an endotracheal tube should be inserted.

Disturbances of respiration

The respiratory centre lies in the lower brain stem (medulla). It is affected in deep coma and also by cerebral herniation. Changes in the rate and rhythm of breathing then occur.

Cheyne–Stokes respiration
This is a periodic form of breathing in which periods of hyperpnoea alternate with periods of apnoea. The hyperpnoeic phases proceed to a crescendo and then decline gradually into apnoea. It is due to an abnormal ventilatory response to carbon dioxide and occurs when the cerebral hemispheres are severely affected in coma of any cause. Its appearance may be a warning of impending herniation.

Central neurogenic hyperventilation
The respiratory rate is rapid and regular and the patient hyperventilates, as reflected by a low arterial P_{CO_2}. It occurs when there is damage to the cerebral hemispheres and upper brain stem.

Ataxic breathing
When the medulla is affected, the respiratory pattern becomes very irregular (ataxic) and respiratory arrest is imminent.

Hypothalamic disturbances

Comatose patients often show some sign of disturbed hypothalamic function. Temperature regulation may be abnormal and the patients temperature increases, often to very high levels. When this happens it is important to exclude other possible causes of a pyrexia.

Regulation of water balance may also be affected, with failure of ADH secretion. The patient then passes large volumes of dilute urine (diabetes insipidus).

The electroencephalogram (EEG) in coma

The EEG records the electrical activity of those layers of the cerebral cortex near to the skull. In comparison to the ECG, it has a much lower voltage (1–100 μV) and is technically more difficult to record. Normally it shows waves of a frequency between 8 and 13 cycles per second (8 and 13 Hz), the alpha rhythm. This frequency slows during sleep.

In coma, various abnormalities may be present in the trace which can be of diagnostic and prognostic value. It may show the presence of a focal lesion if the changes are restricted to a localized area of the skull, whilst in coma due to extrinsic causes, diffuse slow wave abnormalities appear in all areas. In a deeply comatose patient the presence of a normal EEG rules out an extrinsic cause.

Other investigations

Lumbar puncture
The withdrawal of cerebrospinal fluid may be extremely hazardous since it can precipitate coning. Its chief value is in the diagnosis of meningitis, encephalitis and subarachnoid haemorrhage.

Radiology
Plain x-rays of the skull may reveal fractures or shifts of a calcified pineal gland. Carotid angiography is essential in patients with subarachnoid haemorrhage.

Computerized axial tomography 'EMI scanning' has greatly widened the scope of neurological investigations and its use may be extremely valuable. At the present time only a few centres have the necessary apparatus.

Prognosis in coma

Many patients in coma will recover completely if the underlying cause can be treated and no permanent cerebral damage has been sustained. In such cases the coma is usually of relatively short duration—hours or days, rather than weeks.

There are, however, a number of patients who, after the initial phase of intensive therapy, remain in coma with signs of adequate brain stem function but little or no evidence of any higher cortical activity. Within this group is becomes necessary, sooner or later, to distinguish those patients who are irreversibly comatose from those who might still make further significant recovery. There are practical and ethical reasons for this because the continued application of intensive therapy to patients who will only survive in what has been described as a 'persistent vegetative state' is inapproprate. It must be made quite clear, however, since unnecessary confusion still exists, that this is not a problem of determining cerebral death and has nothing to do with the emotive issue of 'switching off a ventilator'. It is simply a question of trying to establish the presence of permanent cerebral damage.

Unfortunately, the prognosis can be extremely difficult to assess because there are no rigid criteria that can be used in an individual patient. General guidelines are the nature and extent of the causative illness, the age of the patient (the young tolerate brain injury better than the elderly) and the duration of the coma. If there are no indications of improvement after one of two weeks, then any meaningful recovery is unlikely. Should improvement, even of a small degree, continue, irrespective of the time scale, then no one at the present time can confidently predict the level of eventual recovery.

Brain death

Throughout history there has been much philosphical debate about the diagnosis of death. Traditionally, death has been accepted to have occurred when the vital functions of respiration and circulation have ceased. The development of intensive therapy with its use of techniques for maintaining ventilation and supporting the circulation has, however, modified these established criteria and has led to the appearance of the syndrome of brain death; in this event all brain function is completely and irreversibly destroyed and the patient is technically dead. No spontaneous breathing is possible and the heart will eventually stop within a matter of hours or days.

The criteria for diagnosing brain death are well established and every ITU must have a clearly defined code of practice for its diagnosis and for discontinuing artificial ventilation. Indecisive management of the situation deprives the patient of death with dignity and needlessly prolongs the distress of the relatives. The morale of the unit staff is also affected if they are required to provide intensive therapy for patients who cannot possibly benefit.

Establishing the presence of brain death is not motivated by the need to provide organs for transplantation; once the diagnosis has been confirmed, however, this clearly has to be considered and, if appropriate, discussed with the patient's relatives.

Causes of brain death

The causes of brain death are:
1. Severe cerebral anoxia, as after a prolonged cardiac arrest.
2. Extensive intracranial haemorrhage.
3. Severe head injuries.

Diagnosis of brain death

If the diagnosis of a disorder which might lead to brain death has been firmly established and the possibility of drugs, hypothermia and endocrine diseases as a cause of the coma have been excluded, the criteria of brain death are:

1. The patient is deeply comatose and maintained on a ventilator because spontaneous breathing has previously stopped.
2. All brain stem reflexes absent:
   - (a) the pupils are fixed in diameter, either widely dilated or in a mid-position, and do not respond to light;
   - (b) the corneal reflex is absent;
   - (c) the occulovestibular, caloric and doll's head reflexes are absent;
   - (d) the cough and gag reflexes are absent;
   - (e) no spontaneous respiratory movements occur when the patient is disconnected from the ventilator for a three minute period, the arterial $P\text{CO}_2$ being normal before disconnection (hypoxia during this time is prevented by giving oxygen through the endotracheal tube or tracheostomy).

   Reflexes of spinal origin, such as flexion to painful stimuli may persist in brain-dead patients.

   The body temperature in patients with cerebral death will fall but should be maintained above 35°C when the above tests are carried out.
3. The EEG is 'flat', showing absence of cerebral electrical activity. Whilst this is not essential for diagnosis, a record should be obtained if an EEG service is available in the hospital.

Cerebral angiography and other methods to demonstrate lack of cerebral blood flow have been used but are unnecessary.

It is customary to repeat all the tests described, to ensure that there has been no observer error. Once this has been completed and the findings confirmed, the patient is declared dead and then ventilatory support is discontinued.

Appendix 1
Normal Values for Adults

Biochemical

Blood

Bilirubin, Total	up to 15 μmol/litre
Calcium, Total	2.20 – 2.55 mmol/litre
Cholesterol, Total	4.0 – 7.0 mmol/litre
Creatinine	45 – 110 μmol/litre
Enzymes:	
Amylase	up to 160 units (Somogyi)
Aspartate aminotransferase (AST)	up to 40 iu/litre
Creatine kinase (CK):	
Males	up to 100 iu/litre
Females	up to 60 iu/litre
γ-Glutamyl transpeptidase (γ-GT):	
Males	6 – 28 iu/litre
Females	4 – 18 iu/litre
2-Hydroxybutyrate dehydrogenase (HBD)	up to 300 iu/litre
5'-Nucleotidase (5-NT)	up to 15 iu/litre
Phosphates: Acid (males only)	up to 5.5 iu/litre
Alkaline (ALKP)	
Males	20 – 85 iu/litre
Females	20 – 70 iu/litre
Glucose (fasting, venous blood)	3.0 – 5.0 mmol/litre
Iodine (protein bound)	310 – 620 nmol/litre
Lactate (fasting, at rest)	0.4 – 1.4 mmol/litre
Magnesium	0.6 – 1.0 mmol/litre
Phosphate	0.6 – 1.3 mmol/litre
Potassium	3.3 – 4.5 mmol/litre
Proteins: Total (plasma)	63 – 81 g/litre
Albumin	36 – 50 g/litre
Globulins (plasma)	24 – 40 g/litre
Sodium	132 – 145 mmol/litre
Urate	0.10 – 0.40 mmol/litre
Urea	3.0 – 7.0 mmol/litre

Urinary Electrolytes

Potassium	35 – 90 mmol/24h
Sodium	100 – 240 mmol/24h
Urea	150 – 500 mmol/24h

Cerebrospinal fluid (Lumbar)

Albumin (immunochemical)	up to 0.4 g/litre
Glucose	3.0 – 4.5 mmol/litre
Protein	0.1 – 0.4 g/litre

Haematological

Haemoglobin:	
Males	13 – 17.5 g/dl
Females	12 – 16.0 g/dl
Packed cell volume (PCV):	
Males	0.40 – 0.50
Females	0.36 – 0.47
Platelet count	150 – 400 × 10^9/litre
Red cell count:	
Males	4.5 – 6.4 × 10^{12}/litre
Females	3.9 – 5.6 × 10^{12}/litre
Reticulocyte count	0.2 – 2%
White cell count:	
Total	4 – 11 × 10^9/litre
Lymphocytes	20 – 45% or 1500 – 3500 × 10^6/litre
Neutrophils	40 – 75% or 2500 – 7500 × 10^6/litre
Sedimentation rate (Westergren)	<10 mm per hour

Appendix 2
Electrolyte composition of some recommended intravenous fluids

Solution	Sodium	Potassium	Chloride	Bicarbonate	Glucose
	(mmol/litre)	(mmol/litre)	(mmol/litre)	(mmol/litre)	(g/litre)
Blood	140	15+	103	0	0
Dextran 40 or 70:					
in 5% dextrose	0	0	0	0	50
in normal saline	144	0	144	0	0
Dextrose 5%	0	0	0	0	50
Dextrose 10%	0	0	0	0	100
Dextrose saline 20% normal saline	31	0	31	0	0
Normal (isotonic) saline	154	0	154	0	0
Packed red cells	10	30+	26	0	0
Plasma	152	15+	100	0	0
Plasma protein fraction (PPF)	150	2	120	0	0
Polygeline (Haemaccel)	145	5	150	0	0
Ringer lactate (Hartmann's)	131	5	112	29 (as lactate)	0
Sodium bicarbonate:					
8.4%	1000	0	0	1000	0
1.5%	178	0	0	178	0

Index